# EMBRACING ALZHEIMER'S

### A Spiritual Journey to Healing the Closed Heart

MARILYN MARCO

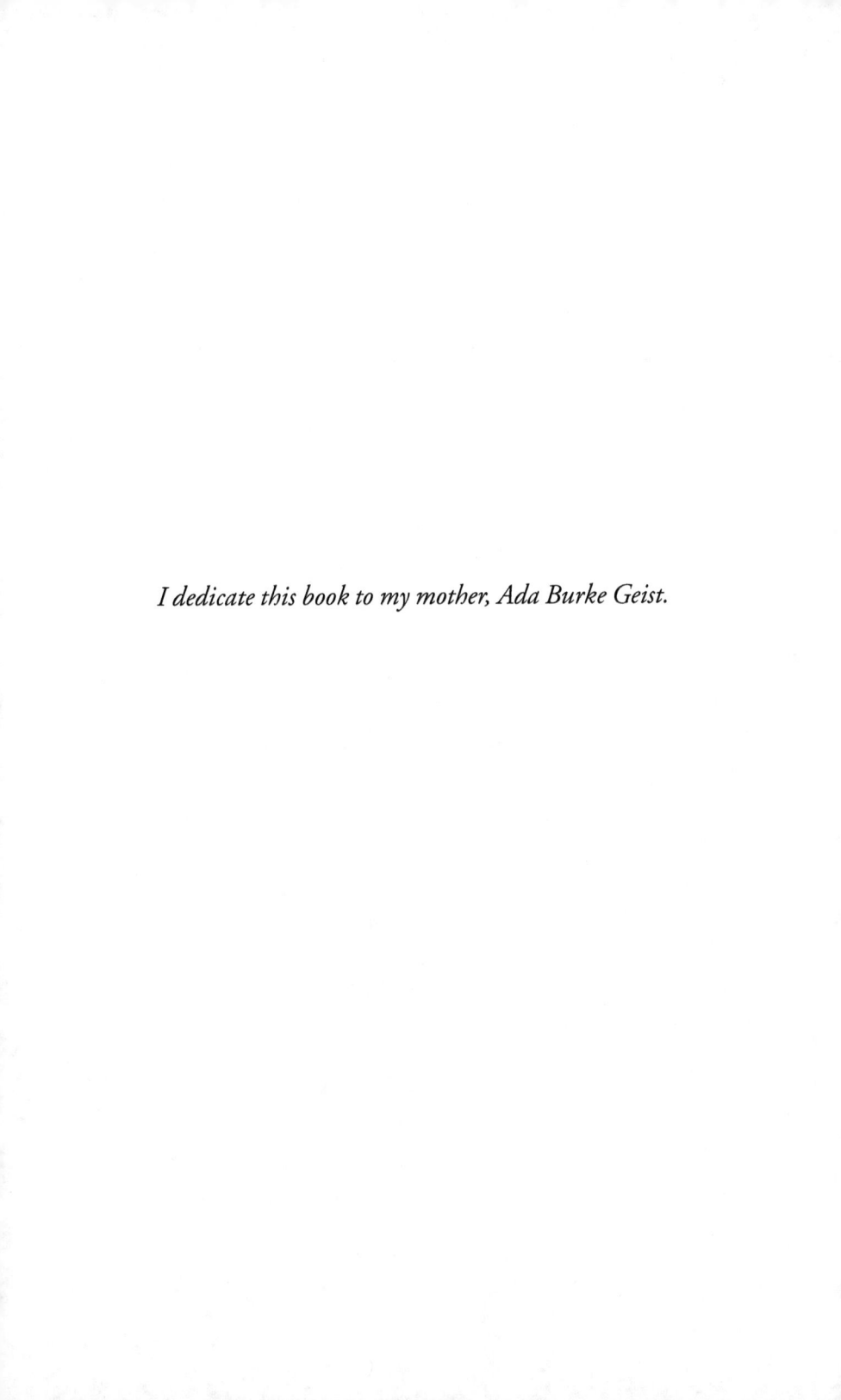

*I dedicate this book to my mother, Ada Burke Geist.*

# Table of Contents

# Introduction

If you have a family member or friend who has Alzheimer's…
or if you're a caregiver for a person who is dealing with it…or
perhaps you're fearful that you might be a candidate for this
disease, I offer this book to give you a roadmap to follow for
prevention, and a pathway to healing that has received little
attention. I have a theory that there is a contributing factor to
Alzheimer's that has not received adequate consideration from
the medical community: the closed emotional heart. With
attention and focused work on the trauma that underlies this
closed heart, it is possible for you and your loved ones to heal
and to claim your birthright to wholeness and health.

I was in danger of closing my heart following a divorce
while also experiencing the devastation of losing my mother
to Alzheimer's. In the midst of these profound challenges, I
had to navigate a fire in my parents' home that threatened
their lives, deal with difficult sibling relationships, and make
hard choices about my mother's care. But it was not until my
maternal grandmother, whom I had never known, came to
me in a channeled communication, that I began my spiritual

journey toward healing and opening my heart. This journey, I believe, saved my life and brought me peace of mind and a clearer sense of purpose.

As a licensed psychotherapist in California with more than 40 years' experience in the mental health field, plus my ongoing private therapy practice of 25 years, I combine offerings from both the fields of psychology as well as spirituality that can guide you on your own healing journey and help open the closed heart. If you are a caregiver, I also offer some guidelines for self-care to follow in order to prevent burnout.

You deserve to have health and happiness in your life – and there is no time to waste. By making some lifestyle changes, paying attention to underlying emotional issues that affect you – and mostly, by making a commitment to the intent to heal yourself – you can put yourself on a path toward living from an open heart. Fueled by your belief that healing is possible, you can achieve a place of peace, and a sense of well-being that has perhaps not yet manifested in your life.

You have gifts to contribute to this world. Let those gifts shine!

# Acknowledgments

I would like to acknowledge the support and excellent editing from Mary Claire Blakeman, who provided constant and invaluable developmental editing skills throughout this whole process.

She was not only extremely knowledgeable and detailed; she was also a great cheerleader, encouraging me to hang in there throughout. I would also like to acknowledge Judi Friedman and Rita Reneaux, who also provided editing suggestions. Jeanne Haynes was my early writing coach, and also storytelling teacher, from whom I received valuable input and training. Her work with me taught me to be in the moment, and taught me how to bring the story to life, both on the page and in live storytelling. My writing support group provided a skilled platform with finely tuned writing skills of their own, from which I drew much encouragement and support.

Thank you to all of you.

# CHAPTER 1

# The Heart Of The Story

Having lived through my mother's Alzheimer's disease, I felt that I had been let into another reality, another world…a world that was not for the faint of heart.

It took me two years of observing and learning about the disease to begin to understand what was going on with my mother. Two years of putting what I had learned together with what I had been told about her strange behaviors to make some sense of it all. My family – like many others coping with this debilitating disease – took much longer to recognize the changes in my mother. They were slow in accepting the fact that these odd behaviors were part of my mother's new reality.

It hit me hard that this person who was acting in ways that were so out of character for her was the mother who took care of me, taught me to care deeply about others less fortunate, taught me to love nature and to name all the flowers, taught me to love learning. Suddenly, I was beginning to live the role reversal, becoming the parent to my mother. It felt like my mother's biggest fear coming true. She had watched her dear paternal grandmother lose her mind, and was fearful all of her life of the same thing happening to her.

For many years after my mother's passing, I felt a strong push to capture the experience I went through and combine it with my background as a psychotherapist of more than forty years to tell another story about this devastating disease.

I wanted to address the critical need for both redefining Alzheimer's and highlighting the deeper meaning of this disease as I experienced it. And, of course, I also wanted to recount some of the funny incidents that happened as I walked with my mother through her Alzheimer's journey. My goal was to offer a book as a vehicle for others to perhaps redefine their own experiences with and fears of Alzheimer's.

My inner motivation to write this book was confirmed when I attended the retirement party for a close friend many years ago. Pat and I had worked together as undergraduate advisers at the University of California, Berkeley, College of Letters and Science, and Pat was retiring from her job. Marian Diamond, PhD, a renowned neuroscientist and one of the founders of modern neuroscience – a professor emerita at U.C. Berkeley who discovered the neuroplasticity of the brain – had been a dean at the College of Letters and Science when I had worked there. I spoke with Dr. Diamond at Pat's retirement party, and told her about my idea to develop a book about my mother's Alzheimer's disease, written from a spiritual and metaphysical point of view – and to portray a different view of the disease, as well as one that included a bit of the lighter side of this difficult experience. Her reply to me was, "Oh, you need to write that book." When a renowned neuroscientist tells you, "…Yes, write that book," you tend to pay attention!

I put off this project for years, and experienced a lack of confidence about it, despite this endorsement from Dr. Diamond. I questioned whether I could really write a book, feared being visible, and allowed my therapy work to occupy my time and energy. It sat neglected on the back burner for many years, but never disappeared.

## Guided from beyond...

While the project languished, something unexpected happened. I began to receive guidance through channeling, also called telepathy. Over the years, this guidance has come to me when I am in meditation, totally quiet, and open to receiving messages and spiritual promptings from angels, guides, relatives, or other divine benevolent beings. It can also occur for me anytime, anywhere – for instance, when I hear "Get off the freeway NOW," which has sometimes steered me away from accidents. This guidance is different from the self-talk we all do throughout our day. It is intuitive communication with any benevolent living or spiritual being that does not rely on the five physical senses.

In spiritual circles, channeling is considered an altered state of consciousness. It involves consciously shifting your mind and mental space in order to achieve an expanded state of consciousness, typically achieved through meditation. The Institute of Noetic Sciences – a nonprofit scientific research center – refers to channeling as "The process of revealing information and energy not limited by space and time."

During meditation, I received channeled communications from my mother Ada, and from her mother, my grandmother Frieda Epstein, whom I never knew. Their messages gave me profound insights into my family's dynamics as well as a unique perspective about my mother's Alzheimer's.

The first time my grandmother came to me was during a meditation when I was doing my own healing work in 2005, following my divorce after an eighteen-year marriage to Jim. I was deeply still when I suddenly felt the clear, powerful presence of Frieda. I had never experienced these sensations before, but I knew clearly that it was her presence.

I had long known the bare outlines of a tragic family story. In my mind and energy field, I heard Frieda recount that story – a tale that involved Frieda's abandoning two of her children, my mother, Ada, age six and her four-year-old brother, Howard. In 1918 Frieda literally put them out on the streets of Philadelphia. She left them alone with lapel tags on their coats saying where their nearest kin lived.

During my meditation, Frieda reframed this dramatic event for me as I heard her say: *"My giving away your mother and her siblings was actually an act of love. I did not have the love in my heart to give them that I knew they needed. And I did not get that love from my mother, and she did not get it from her mother, and that goes back for generations."*

She then paused and said, *"And this MUST stop with you. YOU MUST open your heart."*

## The closed heart...

After receiving the channeled message from my grandmother that I needed to open my heart, I began to focus on my healing in earnest. The message from Frieda led me to examine not only the deep places where I had erected buffers around my own emotions, but to consider how a closed heart affects us all – especially those with Alzheimer's.

I developed a theory, based on all my observations, readings, and therapeutic work, that there is another contributing factor to Alzheimer's disease that has not been adequately addressed: the closed emotional heart.

Underneath the closed heart is unresolved trauma, hurt and pain, often from early childhood experiences; but it can also be a result of trauma suffered as an adult. That trauma can be healed with work on oneself from many sources such as spiritual practices, psychotherapy, somatic body work, meditation, deep self-examination, and mostly a belief that healing can occur – and it is your birthright!

The message that healing of the heart can occur feels ever more important, particularly as the number of aging Baby Boomers reaches a critical mass and our health care system struggles to keep up with the increase in cases of Alzheimer's.

## Heartbreaks and healing...

As I took in the information shared through this channeled message from my grandmother, Frieda, I did not even realize my heart was closed. I had buffered myself from feeling the deep hurt and the loss of my marriage, shoring up my heart from loneliness and fear of allowing in these feelings. To some extent, I had also put aside the memories of how my mother's Alzheimer's may have been inextricably linked with the stress and tension in my marriage.

Intuitively, I knew that my divorce from Jim was the best thing for both of us, as we were on very divergent life paths at the time. Nevertheless, I felt diminished, less desirable, and that, in some way, I had failed. I felt lonely and self-protective.

These feelings were compounded by the fact that I did not have the children I had wanted and was still mourning that loss. I had lost myself in the process of following my husband's dream. When we married in 1987, I had agreed to go cruising the oceans with Jim, in the 37- foot sailboat that he had built. I loved the cruising lifestyle too, but I had unfulfilled dreams of my own. After arriving in Hawaii in 1990 following two years of cruising, I had expected to then start a family. This did not happen, despite efforts that included a round of IVF. I fell into a severe depression but eventually knew I had to bring myself up out of those depths. Deep within me I heard a voice saying, *"You have a choice. You can either become a bitter resentful woman, or you can choose to come up out of these depths and live life with purpose and love."*

I knew my choice was clear. I chose life.

This poem came to me in my later self-healing work, reminding me of my strength.

## YOU ARE

On solitary wings
Do I come to you
I breathe into your soul
I light your eyes
I rustle the leaves
And the wind blows
Away your tears.
You are rooted in earth
The stones hear you
The woods are alive
With your cries and sighs.
Your heart is so deep
Your sensitivities
So translucent
You are wired to everything
All at once.

Though I had come out of my depression, the disappointment about not starting a family remained. The tension between my desires and the pull of the ocean for my seafaring husband grew stronger. Those years in the early 1990s marked the beginning of a crisis in our marriage.

It was soon after I made the choice to embrace love instead of becoming bitter, that I knew I needed to make a major shift in my life. At that point, my mother's Alzheimer's took a downward turn, and my father was suddenly hospitalized with life threateningly high blood sugar levels. This crisis for my parents necessitated my taking an emergency flight to San Francisco from Hawaii where we were living, and to make plans to care for both my mother and father for six weeks. Becoming a caretaker for my mother with Alzheimer's at this time somewhat filled my need for nurturing – but it did not stop the downward spiral of our marriage. Once the immediate crisis with my parents' health settled down a bit, I rejoined Jim in Hawaii. Not long afterwards, in 1994, we sailed back to the San Francisco Bay Area where Jim and I eventually moved off of our sailboat and began living on land once again.

Jim waited for me for years to be ready to go cruising again. Though I loved that life as well, I finally told him that he needed to go, as sailing was his lifeblood and passion and I didn't want to keep him from that. And I knew there were things that I needed to do at home in California. Those things turned out to be my own healing and development of my spiritual path, as well as engaging in further professional development as a family therapist.

We finally divorced in 2005 so that we could have a clean break with the understanding that we could each pursue other relationships if we so chose. I should note here that Jim and I remained connected, despite our divorce. We have an enduring deep love and connection that has remained over decades, but a connection that has allowed for other relationships. Over the ensuing years, we both traveled back and forth to be with each other in California, as well as Tonga and Fiji, where Jim lived on his boat for many years. In June 2024, he came to live with me permanently at my invitation, after I experienced a palpable divine intervention that led me to ask him to return home from Fiji to live with me. While that is our story now, there is much more of the story of my mother's life and mine to tell.

## The roots of Alzheimer's

Years ago, I spent a great deal of time trying to understand how such a brilliant and healthy woman as my mother could have acquired Alzheimer's. Her mind was perpetually in motion, her body was constantly on the move with many projects and daily walking in the neighborhood. Her diet was excellent and she made everything from scratch. No processed foods or even excess sugar. She had an occasional drink but didn't overdo it. She had many friends and was active in numerous groups.

I began to see the connection between my mother's closed heart stemming from her early life trauma, possibly resulting in Alzheimer's in her later life. I saw her slide into a younger state of mind, one that held the ideal of being safely held as a young vulnerable soul.

As I struggled to understand how this devastating disease could so drastically attack someone like my mother, I began to explore the research about Alzheimer's. Much work on the causes of Alzheimer's has been done, and more continues to be revealed about this disease. Yet there is no cure, and no reliable, affordable medication has been developed. There are however, warnings from neuroscientists of 'cascading' Alzheimer's risk from two habits. While they acknowledge that the risk is dependent on a range of genetic and environmental factors – and genes may have played a role in my mother's condition as she feared "losing her mind" like her paternal grandmother – the two most impactful causes of Alzheimer's are alcohol consumption and chronic stress, according to Nikki Crowley, director of the Penn State Neuroscience Institute and an assistant professor of biology.

In my therapy practice, I see the effects of chronic stress in particular, and the toll it takes on my clients' health, life, and relationships. This chronic stress eats away at a person's sense of well-being and can undermine their ability to achieve goals in life. A high level of alcohol consumption is also detrimental to a healthy, self-fulfilled life. Combined together, these two factors greatly increase the risk for Alzheimer's, as well as other health risks.

However, I have not observed research that gives adequate attention to Adverse Childhood Experiences (ACEs) as a contributing cause of Alzheimer's. "Frontiers in Aging

Neuroscience" – a leading journal in the field of research on the biological processes of human aging – published an article in 2022 acknowledging the fact that few studies have examined the relationship between adverse events early in life and Alzheimer's. The article, however, does report that chronic stress throughout the adult lifespan has been consistently associated with a decline in cognitive function, and an increased risk of dementia. Other research through the National Institutes of Health cites a study conducted by Kayla B. Corney in 2022 on "The Relationship Between Adverse Childhood Experiences and Alzheimer's Disease: A Systematic Review." This study states that "adverse childhood experiences may increase the risk of developing Alzheimer's disease." But it concludes by saying that further research is needed.

Our nation is brimming with a population that has been traumatized in many ways. From childhood abuse and neglect, to the experience of millions who grow up in alcoholic and toxic families, to the continuing negative effects from the Covid pandemic that resulted in so many deaths, to the Fentanyl crisis and many other negative national events, we are a country that is hurting. Since the end of the pandemic, the field of mental health appears to have lost some of its stigma around the idea of seeking help for personal emotional issues. In my therapy practice, I am seeing more men than in the past, particularly post pandemic. More and more men are opening up and asking, "Why am I feeling depressed or stuck in life? Why are my relationships not working? What can I do to feel better about myself and my direction in life?" And, they are willing to look into past family history and previous dysfunctional relationships to discover what has kept them stuck in repetitive cycles.

I am also seeing many more couples than in the past. They too are wanting to delve into their unproductive patterns of communication and dissatisfaction. They are more willing to look at the underlying causes of their discontent – such as blaming their partners and not taking responsibility for what they bring to the table, withholding communication, and neglecting to express appreciation and respect for each other.

Over the years I have worked with abused and neglected children removed from their families and placed in foster care. I have also worked in the court system mediating between parents fighting over custody of their children, and have been responsible for conducting thorough investigations to determine and recommend to the court the best custody arrangements for a child or siblings. This work revealed the origins of many mental health issues to me, as well as the damage inflicted on children and families who are involved in the court system and public agencies. It was very difficult work, but excellent training.

What I see with many clients in my private therapy practice are hearts that have been protected – and sometimes closed – from childhood. Perhaps they developed this emotional armor due to those early adverse experiences, combined with poor parental models of dealing with emotions. Often, there is also an effort to avoid looking at what is underneath the trauma, pain, or general discontent. This self-protection is most often unconscious. What is lacking is the realization that it compromises their current relationships and functioning, and often results in repetitive unsatisfying communication and behavior patterns. What I also see are attempts to fill the internal emptiness with addictions to any number of things such as alcohol, drugs, sex, or constant acquisition of material things. The heart is closed and does not want to feel the trauma that is underneath. This is a survival mechanism put in place from a young age. With 40 years of experience in my profession, I know it is critical for therapists to have compassion and honesty in working with such clients.

In the course of providing couples therapy, I have witnessed over and over the impact of closed hearts in so many of these relationships. Often, in a heterosexual relationship it is the man who is unable to access his feelings and to express his emotions, which leaves the woman wanting more and feeling empty. This is not surprising, given the cultural training boys and men receive from a young age to not show "weakness" by crying, or exhibiting their soft sides, or being in touch with their vulnerabilities. Their humanity and sensitivities are trained out of them to the point where their hearts and souls suffer. Women can exhibit the same difficulties with accessing the expression of emotions in a healthy manner, and can also have difficulty in opening up honestly. We learn from our parents/guardians first, and most of us from the Boomer generation did not learn to be honest about and express our feelings. In my family, emotions were not discussed, but were acted out in unhealthy ways. It was not until I went away to college and began to be in serious relationships that I learned to express my feelings. I had to learn how to communicate on my own, but once I did, it opened up the well of emotions that I didn't know I had been missing.

## The path that led to my mother's Alzheimer's

My experiences – both personal and professional – coupled with what I learned from researchers about Alzheimer's gave me insights about my mother and how such a vibrant person developed this disease.

Clearly, being abandoned on the street in Philadelphia at age six was a trauma that shaped my mother and reverberated throughout her life. I see this early trauma as the core cause of her closing a part of her heart. I believe her closed heart – as well as the experience of spending a lifetime in a typical 1950s marriage with a controlling man – were contributing factors in my mother's Alzheimer's diagnosis.

Additionally, she suppressed the dreams she had for her life. She loved to sing and played the piano, and perhaps thought of pursuing that interest. Instead, my older sister, Louise, lived out that dream for her by moving to Vienna, Austria and studying to become an opera singer, allowing my mother to at least, for a time, vicariously realize her fantasies through my sister. I now realize that depression was also a major factor that contributed to my mother's Alzheimer's.

Typical of the era of the 1950s and 1960s, my mother had a medicine cabinet well stocked with a variety of medicines, including a barbiturate prescribed by her doctor, perhaps as an anti-depressant, perhaps for pain. When that doctor retired and she had to change to another, she assumed she would be able to continue with her prescription for Phenobarbital, but was brusquely told, "I never prescribe that for my patients." My mother seemed surprised at this pronouncement from the doctor, but as far as I know, she did not have problems with stopping this medication. I simply don't recall hearing anything dramatic about this change in her prescriptions.

What I do know, however, is that she was good at learning about whatever ailed her and attempting anything that might help. For instance, I remember when I was in college in the early 1970s, my mother read Norman Cousins' groundbreaking book, "*Anatomy of An Illness*", on combating life-threatening illness through using humor to boost the bodies' capacity for self-healing. This led to her reading more books of humor and comedy. In the same vein, she also read Bernie Siegal's "*Love, Medicine and Miracles*" around that time. This book outlines the healing power of unconditional love and was an early guide to self-healing through using the power of one's mind. Indeed, my mother was an early role model for me in pursuing my interest in self-healing.

In later conversations with my father, he related something that my mother kept repeating to him when she was in the early stages of Alzheimer's: "I feel like I'm losing my mind!" For someone as intellectual and brilliant as my mother, this had to be terrifying! She was indeed, losing her mind, her most precious and valuable asset. As I have tried to imagine over the years what that must have been like, the fear grabs me at the throat and shakes me to my core. My father later recounted to me, that when my mother was in the grip of that terror, he didn't know what to do. He would end up phoning her best friend, Evelyn, and ask that she come over to be with my mother. When I asked Evelyn about these episodes later, she told me, "I didn't know what to do. The only thing that would somewhat work was to give her a drink." Well, at least someone had found a temporary cure.

These experiences must have been terrifying for my father as well, as he began to watch the steady deterioration of his life partner, the gradual disappearance of the woman he had known, and to grieve daily for the wife he loved so much.

In observing my father, I realized I was also witnessing his transformation from a controlling though doting husband who failed to recognize my mother's emotional needs in their earlier years, to a husband who was in the throes of daily grieving, as he witnessed my mother's intellectual essence ebb away as she became a shell of herself. He was losing his beloved wife day by day, never knowing how long this disease would last, or what trajectory her decline would follow. In the course of this journey, my father softened and his loving, caring, tender side grew tremendously.

I had always been the favored child in the family, and had an easier relationship with my father than my siblings. I think he had also come to respect my expertise in the mental health field, and turned to me for help in understanding both my mother and my sister. Consequently, he leaned on me for support and guidance, for comfort and solace. He had softened greatly in this most difficult stage of life, and looked to me for support that was available nowhere else.

As I supported my parents through all the ups and downs of life and the difficult stages of Alzheimer's, I continued to struggle with the question of why this disease had so devastated the mind of my brilliant mother. The medical research gave me some insights, but I knew I would have to look beyond it for the answers I sought. As a therapist, I understood the value of examining the past – but I knew only fragments of my mother's history.

I knew I would have to search my mother's past to get to the heart of the story.

# CHAPTER 2

# My Newly Discovered Grandparents

I am a child about ten years old. I am sitting at the kitchen table after the rest of the family has finished dinner and left. My mother is busy cleaning up and washing dishes. I want to ask her some important questions that have been on my mind.

"*Mom, what is our ethnic background?*"

My mother stiffens and stops her cleaning. She gazes straight ahead, and says, "Why do you ask?"

"*Because I know about Daddy's German background, but not about your background.*"

She pauses, and then in a strong voice says, "Well, we're a little English, a little German, and a little Russian Jew."

It is that last part, "a little Russian Jew" that fascinates me the most, and I want to know about it. But my mother would only answer basic questions about her mother. Her protective wall was always up and I knew even as a child not to push her too far.

What I really wanted to ask was, "How could your mother leave you and your brother on the streets? How could she get rid of her kids like that?" I never asked those questions, but I couldn't stop wondering about it. The whole thing made no sense to my 10-year-old mind.

My mother would tell me that her mother was a very self-centered person, and a hypochondriac who would play on people's sympathies for attention. It was later in my career as a therapist that I realized my grandmother carried the diagnosis of Narcissistic Personality Disorder.

My mother did tell me this part of the story: Her older sister, Helen, stayed with their mother, Frieda, for a time after my mother and her brother Howard were abandoned on the streets in Philadelphia.

Since Helen was older, she could do work for Frieda, around the house, presumably. Helen was later sent to Wyoming where my mother and her brother also ultimately ended up. They were first taken to an orphanage for the night after being abandoned by Frieda, and then sent by train to their father in Idaho. However, their father, George, quickly realized he could not take care of three young children, and asked his two sisters who lived on the ranch in Wyoming if they would take them. Yes, of course they would. So, the children were all sent to their aunt Julia and aunt Bessie, on the large ranch near La Grange, Wyoming, where they were raised.

I am about twenty years old, visiting my Uncle Howard, my mother's brother, and his wife Vernice. Howard tells me, "There is something I want to tell you that I know your mother will never tell you." In my mind, I am gleefully rubbing my hands together, "Oh, boy, what is it? You can always count on my Uncle Howard for the family dirt!"

Howard proceeds to tell me, "You are one quarter Jewish."

*"Well, I know that. Mom never made a secret of it, but she always told us we are one-eighth Jewish."*

"No," Howard went on, "Our mother's name was Epstein, and she was full Jewish. That makes us one half Jewish, and makes you one quarter."

Somehow, this revelation from my uncle hit home with me, and I suddenly felt my Jewish heritage for the first time in my heart! It explained so much about me to myself. It explained why I had so many Jewish friends. It explained my social, cultural and political interests.

I suddenly felt more complete, and I let out a joyful "Shalom!" But one day, I went back to my mother and asked her, "Hey, what about this? Howard says we are one quarter Jewish." She answered me in a very curt, indignant tone, "I don't know where he gets that. It's only one eighth." My mother's denial of her Jewish heritage was glaring, but in my early 20s, I didn't really understand the full import of her feelings.

Another piece of the story comes from something my mother *did* speak about openly. She attended the University of Wyoming in Laramie. In order to get into the sorority of her choice, she had to sign a paper that stated "I have no Jewish blood." Even today, in our culture which remains racist and anti-Semitic, this requirement is shocking. However, at that time, in the early 1930's, it is important to remember Nazism was very much at hand and identifying as Jewish would have been a reason for being ostracized, or perhaps even put in danger.

It is apparent that my mother's denial of her Jewish heritage had several roots. One of those roots, and the most important, I believe, was the painful and traumatic abandonment on the streets by her mother, Frieda, which led to the erasure of her mother from her consciousness. And two, the political climate of the time demanded that my mother deny her Jewish heritage.

As I came to know more of the complexity of my grandmother's life, I realized that she was a brilliant woman who came from a brilliant family. Frieda accepted a job in Camaguey, Cuba in the early 1900's, working as an interpreter for Abbott Laboratories after having been a teacher for some years in the U.S. Camaguey is in the central part of Cuba and is now the third largest city on the island. She would have landed this job through her father, Dr. Ephraim Epstein, who was a well-known and accomplished man in many fields, being a physician, a theologian, a minister, a linguist who spoke seven languages, and a scholar. Obviously, the lingual ability that runs through my ancestors, and my own family of origin, had been passed on to my grandmother.

Her father was well connected to the founder of Abbott Laboratories. Frieda would have met her husband, George Harvey Burke, an American cowboy from Idaho, in Camaguey, a city known for cattle raising. George was also in Cuba because he had gone there as part of future president Teddy Roosevelt's Rough Riders. That name was given to the First U.S. Volunteer Cavalry, a regiment of about one thousand men that included a diverse mix of Native Americans, athletes, miners, Texas Rangers and others who served in the Spanish American War in Cuba in 1898.

My grandparents, Frieda Epstein and George Harvey Burke, married in Camaguey in 1909. From family lore, confirmation from my aunt Joan Yates, as well as channeled communications from my grandmother, Frieda, it is clear that George was a dashing, handsome, wild cowboy who was the complete opposite of Frieda's intellectual, accomplished and strict father, Ephraim Epstein. The sparks flew when they met. In this channeled communication from my grandmother, Frieda related more of what attracted her to George Harvey Burke:

*"It was his sense of adventure that also drew me to him. Yes, he was very handsome, his eyes deep and soulful. But his depth of feeling drew me in – lost in his arms and embrace, it felt like the all-encompassing love from a man that I had missed with my*

*father. My father was not warm and embracing. He was distant, not available, stuck "in his head" as you would say.*

*George was so the opposite of my father. I longed for adventure and color in my life, and for escape…escape to another world, free of all the restrictions and constrictions I felt. George had a softness in his eyes, a vulnerability I had never seen before in a man's eyes. And a laugh! He had a wonderfully boisterous, infectious laugh that filled me with delight. I had never experienced that in my life. I felt I was exploring new frontiers of my being I had never before experienced. And he introduced me to nature, horses, and the wild outdoors.*

*That was all new for me. It excited me no end. But this was short lived, as it was no more than three or four months after our wedding that he was again roving his eyes over all the women. My infatuation made for great sex. But there were many beautiful, sensual women to behold in Cuba. With the arrival of our first child, Helen, things briefly perked up. A baby seemed to initially bring him back to me. However, Helen was a colicky baby, difficult to soothe or calm. This seemed to drive George out again. And I was engulfed by Helen's needs."*

My aunt Helen was their first child, born in 1911. My mother was born one year later, in 1912. When I was perhaps in my teens, my older sister mentioned that Helen was born with syphilis. I wondered how she knew this, but my sister being four years older than I, knew things I did not. It seems the obvious explanation for why my aunt Helen was so sickly all of her life, and always appeared many years older than she was. George was quite the philanderer, a known family fact. Another confirmed fact was that he died in a Veterans Administration home in Arizona of syphilis.

From what I know from family stories and what I received in Frieda's messages, my sense is that my grandmother wanted out of her constricted life in the U.S. – and Cuba represented an opportunity and an exotic escape to another land. In one of my channelings from Frieda, this message came through:

*"In the shadow of my father and even my mother, who was quite formidable, I felt small. I felt less than I should be. Expectations in this family were high. I chafed under the strict rules, longed to be free, longed to be my own rule setter. This is why George so caught my attention, and my heart, in the beginning. He was wild and free! ...as I longed to be. Yet I also wanted to please my father and mother, wanted them to approve of me, wanted their love."*

At another time, I received this additional message from my grandmother:

*"I wanted out of my staid life. I wanted to see other lands, have new experiences, and experience more of life. My father was glad to arrange for me to meet with Mr. Miley, from Abbott Labs. Perhaps if I had met with Dr. Abbott himself, I would not have been offered the job. I used my brains and beauty to convince Mr. Miley to accept me into the Abbott family. I was well qualified. I spoke Hebrew, German and some Spanish. I was very intelligent in math, English and the sciences. I was well read and well bred. I was a hard worker, had strict ethics and morals, and was reliable and punctual. And I was willing to take risks and go to foreign lands."*

After receiving this message and some time had passed, I realized that my grandmother was a woman ahead of her time because she had a serious career. Children interfered with her career, and as the narcissist she was, perhaps she never really wanted children.

And Frieda's message did not stop with her explanation of how she landed the job at Abbott Labs. She continued with this description of Cuba:

*"I was dizzy with the newness of Cuba when I first arrived. The colors, the sights and sounds, the lush landscape, the freedom with which people gave themselves over to music, dance, language and dress. I was a foreigner in a foreign land, yet something felt so familiar and comforting to me. Yes, I did mostly commune only with Americans, but the Cubans were very accessible."*

In 2016, I met a cousin in London, Susan Lee Kerr, whom I did not know of until my sister-in-law, Else, in Norway discovered her on the internet. Else was very interested in our family genealogy and found out that Susan, a writer, journalist, and artist, had published a book, *"The Extraordinary Dr. Epstein"* after doing fifteen years of research. Dr. Ephraim Epstein is Susan's and my great grandfather. Susan's grandmother and my grandmother, Frieda, were sisters. Susan had been looking for descendants of Ephraim Epstein on the internet when my sister-in-law found her, and I wrote an email to Susan introducing myself. When I visited her in London at her home, it felt like we had known each other all our lives.

As I learned from Susan and her book, Ephraim Epstein immigrated to the U.S. in 1850 from Belarus, Russia, when he was nineteen years old. He grew up in a very rigid Orthodox Jewish family that did not allow reading outside of the Torah. With his superior intelligence, he chafed under this harsh and uncompromising upbringing, as he wanted to learn all he could about the world. In later years in the U.S., Ephraim converted to Christianity and became a minister, and he replicated the restrictive environment of his Orthodox family. Consequently, my grandmother was raised in her father's very strict Christian home, where each child was expected to read from the Bible before meals.

My grandmother Frieda was the third child of Ephraim and his wife, Helena. The tragic and unexpected death of their first-born child, William, at age four, threw Ephraim into a deep depression and numbed state, which apparently lasted several years. During this depression, their second born child, Selda, died unexpectedly at age two. I cannot even begin to imagine the depth of this pain and loss for both Ephraim and his wife. Perhaps it was this depression that caused my grandmother to proclaim her father was "distant and unavailable" in one of the channeled communications I received from her. Additionally, with the deaths of the first two children in the family, Frieda became the eldest of seven children. That position would have put a burden on her of being held as the responsible eldest, and most likely led to her having to care for her younger siblings. Perhaps later in life this burden was also a source of her apparent resentment of her own children's needs.

I am moved to note here the connections I see between my grandmother Frieda's passions, as well as what attracted her to George, and myself. My husband, Jim, was the one who introduced me to sailing and cruising the high seas. Travel has always been one of my passions, but I never envisioned sailing the oceans. Though I was terrified at the prospect, there was something in Jim that called forth the risktaker in me, the wild adventurer, willing to leave everything known and familiar and predictable in my life in the Bay Area of San Francisco, for the unknown. Somehow, I simply trusted Jim from a very deep place in my soul. He became my master sailing teacher, but also opened me up to life experiences I never would have had otherwise, and tapped into a confidence and skill at mastering new vistas that I couldn't have dreamed of or thought possible. Jim also has the softness of soul and willingness to be vulnerable that perhaps my grandfather George showed to my grandmother Frieda.

The connections between my grandparent's relationship and mine with Jim are striking to me. I wondered how else my family's story would intertwine with ours and impact our relationship. I was soon to find out.

# CHAPTER 3

# A Ride on the Downward Slide

My husband Jim, and I arrive in Tahiti in the summer of 1990 on our 37-foot sailboat after cruising around the waters of Mexico for a year and a half, including living in Zihuatanejo for three months. After a 24-day sail across the Pacific, we then spend another two months exploring the Marquesas Islands and part of the Tuamotus Archipelago of French Polynesia. Arriving in Tahiti – the largest and most developed island in French Polynesia – we receive a bounty of mail for the first time in months. Opening these letters always feels like Christmas for us, when we get to read several months of letters from family and friends.

There is a letter from my father, written about a month previously. I open it excitedly to hear of their news, but am taken aback as my father is asking me to come home because my mother had suffered some period of disorientation and confusion. With my brow furrowing in worry, I sink into the cushion as I take in this concerning news. I tell Jim I have to find a phone and call home to figure out what is going on. I feel the urgency and trepidation as I make my way to the shore in search of a landline phone I can use. First, I call one of my parents' best friends, Bill, who was also our former family physician, to ask if indeed, I actually need to return home. The doctor and his wife, Evelyn, tell me my mother had gone through some kind of period of disorientation. But, she appeared to be fine now and I did not need to return home. They relate to me how my mother suddenly could not follow their usual bridge game that they and my parents had been playing regularly for years. I feel relieved to hear I do not need to go home, but confused as to what exactly is going on.

I then phone my mother from Tahiti, but because I am paying $10 a minute for the call and we are on a very tight budget, I ask my mother to call me back. She sounds like herself, but in trying to give her the phone number at which to reach me, she becomes very confused and can't understand the numbers I'm giving her. I didn't know it at the time, but this difficulty with numbers and simple arithmetic is one of the early signs of Alzheimer's. As I put the phone back on the receiver, I lean against the wall and am suddenly reeling from my first encounter with my mother's slide into Alzheimer's. This was my mother, the brilliant math major, the community activist, and master organizer of details who ran the English Department at Chico State! And she's confused about a simple phone number!

I consult two fellow cruising friends who are physicians, and describe to them what I knew at that point, as well as the difficult phone call with my mother. Carol says, "It sounds like it might be early dementia." Dementia!

Even though I am a trained psychotherapist, I had not encountered this diagnosis and was only vaguely familiar with it. Suddenly, my heart drops with the first glimmer into the beginning of my mother's Alzheimer's disease.

Though I was shaken by the phone call, I was assured by our family friends that I did not need to rush back to the states. Jim and I stayed in French Polynesia for several more months before sailing to Hawaii in late 1990. We established ourselves in Honolulu in residence on the boat, and secured jobs in our fields. Jim initially taught sailing, and then was First Mate on a large dinner/disco cruise boat off of Waikiki, while I worked as a program manager in a child abuse prevention program.

In our first year in Hawaii, I followed a friend around town as she visited her father-in-law who had Alzheimer's. It was then that I began to learn about the symptoms of the disease first hand. In his house I saw the hand written notes attached to appliances, with instructions on how to operate them. This experience was a major turning point. After close to a year of accompanying my friend on those visits to her father-in-law, I suddenly realized that my mother probably had Alzheimer's.

I went to the office of the Alzheimer's Association in Honolulu and picked up their literature. I compared what I knew of my mother's behavior and symptoms to the list of symptoms in the literature – difficulty with numbers and simple arithmetic, decline of social skills, social withdrawal, inability to follow her favorite card game of bridge, getting lost trying to find her way back from the hairdresser, and subsequently giving up her driver's license voluntarily. Even my husband told me that at the time of our marriage four years earlier, he noticed that my mother was not tracking conversations.

I had not been aware of this at the time, but family members are often the ones who don't see Alzheimer's symptoms early on, either due to their closeness of relationship, or denial, or both. When I look at photos taken of my mother in those early years, I can see evidence of the Alzheimer's. She is withdrawn, her body slumping inward, her face looking shy and blank. This was not who my mother was. She was normally a gregarious, socially-engaged and outgoing person.

While Jim and I were living in Hawaii and I came to realize that my mother had Alzheimer's, I began writing to my father, sister and brother, to alert them to my concerns about my mother. What I ran into was their denial. "No, she doesn't have Alzheimer's," was their response. One reason a person can "pass" for a long time among family members and close friends was exhibited by my mother. She was not generating ideas of her own and she was not taking initiative in regard to projects, ideas or plans. But, she was good at spouting platitudes that sounded close enough to something she would say, for example, "You can't judge a book by its cover", or tacking on agreement to something someone else had said, but not adding her own thoughts.

For two years, while my family continued stonewalling the problem, I persisted in outlining her symptoms and my concerns. I urged my father to take my mother for a medical consultation. Finally, around 1992, when my mother was 80 years old, my father took her in for an exam. That's when my mother was diagnosed with Alzheimer's. In looking back, however, I realize that her disease probably started at least five to seven years earlier. Scientists and medical experts now state that Alzheimer's symptoms actually begin to appear approximately twenty years before an official diagnosis.

It's 1994 and Jim and I are still living in Hawaii. The phone rings. It's Evelyn, my mother's best friend, giving me this urgent message: "Marilyn, you're going to need to get over here as soon as possible. Your father is in the hospital with dangerously high blood sugar levels. A county worker is caring for your mother at home until you can get here."

My heart drops and fear suddenly grips me. I feel frantic. My mother had already reached a point in her downhill slide where she could not be left alone. I tell Jim I have to get back home immediately. I fly out to San Francisco two days later and stay six weeks in the northern California town of Paradise in my childhood home. My mother seems relieved to see me, but confused. She does not quite understand what is happening and wonders where my father is. I had been waiting for a crisis to develop, knowing that my father would not let me make any arrangements for my mother to get the care that she needed without an intervening crisis such as the emergency of his own stay in the hospital. I realized he could revert to his overcontrolling ways and desire to protect my mother as her only caretaker. Only later, as my mother's disease progressed, did he begin to accept more help. I witnessed his unflagging support for her continue to grow and soften as the loving, caring spouse he was.

Recognizing the dynamics at play in my family, I take advantage of this crisis point to place my mother in a wonderful day program I find in Paradise. It's a part-time program that she can attend for three half days per week. This small group program has about eight to ten people, all suffering the early to mid-stages of Alzheimer's. It offers many wonderful activities specifically geared for their condition, such as singing and other musical activities, recalling and telling of past fond memories or personal stories, playing word games, engaging in movement exercises, and developing creative art projects. What is most striking to me, is that the people in the program recognize their similar disabilities, and bond with each other around those commonalities. They speak each other's language.

At the end of the first day of the program, I drive to pick up my mother. After she climbs into the passenger seat, I ask her, "So how was it?" Her answer is both gut-wrenching and reassuring to me, "I feel human again!" She is giddy with happiness, and my heart soars. I realize then, that the slide into the darkness of Alzheimer's must feel like losing one's humanness, and all that defines us as an individual. What a terrifying slide, indeed.

These experiences must have been terrifying for my father as well, as he began to watch the steady deterioration of his life partner, the gradual disappearance of the woman he had known, and to grieve daily for the wife he loved so much, despite their flawed marriage.

At the time, I didn't really know how the day program was affecting my mother. It was only after my trips to Cuba in later years, when I began receiving frequent channeled communications from her, that I started to understand its impact on her life.

Here is one of her channeled messages to me:

*"It is a terrifying disease that made me feel I was losing not only my mind, but my soul and my humanity. I was grateful when you took me to the day care center. It is important to be with others who also have Alzheimer's. We can relate to each other, feel each other, and know we are not alone. Music, and reading of literature and poetry also helped immensely... music especially, because it so transported me past my mind, past my fears and feelings of numbness and deadness. It tapped into my heart!"*

My mother was able to capitalize on her skills in this small group program in Paradise, another win for her. With her superior language, writing and grammar skills, when reading aloud or doing word games in the group, my mother was able to shine. The program director commented on this to me and was quite impressed with my mother's ability.

Another thing happened in this program: my mother's long-lost flirtatiousness resurfaced. There was a man in the group that my mother took a particular liking to, and apparently did not try to hide her interest in him. I'm not sure how that played out in the group, but the program directors were well aware of this development. One day I asked my mother, "Mom, how old do you think you are?" "Sixteen," she immediately responded. And yes, she was acting just like a very flirtatious sixteen-year-old. Indeed, my mother seemed to be losing most of her inhibitions.

It is well known among staff in programs of residential Alzheimer's patients, that the boundaries of sexual behavior and flirtation can be very blurred. A few years later, when I was checking out Alzheimer's living facilities for my mother in the city of Chico, not too far from Paradise, a staff member at one facility told me that the residents on the locked unit would freely roam between their rooms, and even help themselves to each other's clothing. What a creative sharing community.

At the end of my six-week stay in Paradise, after I had gotten my mother into the day program and my father's health had stabilized somewhat, I told my husband Jim that I would need to return to California in order to take care of my parents. This announcement led to a critical crossroads in our relationship, as Jim wanted to stay in Hawaii. I made it clear that I was going to return to California whether he came with me or not.

Ultimately, we weathered the storm and made plans for sailing back to California in the summer of 1994. We arrived in San Francisco on a clear night after a 21-day sail, cruising in under the Golden Gate Bridge, accompanied by our close sailing friend Richard who came to meet us in his boat. Richard had been the friend who was also with us on his boat on our original cruising departure under the same Golden Gate five and a half years earlier. What a glorious homecoming it was, with a calm sea and a moon shining down upon us!

That calm didn't last, however. The next few years were tumultuous and unpredictable. Jim and I lived on and off our boat, with several different friends, but eventually I informed him that I was moving to an apartment as I needed to be land based. Reluctantly, the hardcore sailor agreed and we moved to an apartment in the town of Alameda, just across the Bay from San Francisco. I was already commuting the three-hour drive back and forth fairly frequently from Alameda to Paradise to see my parents and assess their situation.

My father's initial health crisis with his high blood sugar levels had passed, and he was able to continue taking care of my mother. After much searching, we found a personal aide who came almost every day to help my mother. And my mother continued in the day program three half days a week. My father finally discovered what a relief it was to have a break from caring for my mother, to get some things done and have a bit of time for himself. He was eventually open to educating himself as well, and acquired the book, "*The 36-Hour Day*", by Nancy Mace, M.A. and Peter Rabins, M.D., M.P.H. In those early stages of my mother's Alzheimer's, we did the best we could – not knowing how many more of those "36-Hour Days" lay ahead of us.

# CHAPTER 4

# Light Shines – Even Through the Darkness of Alzheimer's

It's 1995 and my mom is in the middle stage of Alzheimer's. My dad and I have navigated through the early stage of terror and paranoia on her part, and sadness, fear, and letting go on ours. One particularly painful period of my mother's paranoia, was when she accused my father and me of conspiring to get her out of the house. "You're trying to get rid of me!", she screams. Her fear and anger are palpable. Simply trying to reassure her that this is not true, does not ease her anxiety and delusional suspicions.

Dad, my mom's lifelong partner, has unflinchingly taken on all the duties my mother used to carry – grocery shopping, meal preparation, bill paying, housecleaning, in addition to being my mom's caregiver. This new, softer version of my father is a role I had not previously witnessed in him, as he had been much more controlling and sometimes abusive to my brother earlier in my life. It is clear that dealing with this disease and watching his wife decline day by day, is changing my father. He doesn't complain. He educates himself about this unforgiving disease, and cries with me at the loss of his beloved wife.

Once my mother got through the early stage of Alzheimer's and was so far gone that she didn't know how far gone she was, she lost the paranoia and terror. She also lost all her tendency to judge and criticize others, and to engage in self-judgment. What emerged was her true essence – her sweetness, her playfulness, and her humor. "There she goes again, speaking 'Ada-ese'," I would say to her, as she spoke the garbled language unique to my mother, Ada. Often, her comments started out fine, but deteriorated into a word salad.

Slowly and painfully, I learned to let go of expectations, let go of ordinary reality, and enter into my mom's world. In doing so, my mother was able to relax, be her new self, and to laugh. Alzheimer's patients' emotions are intact and they are highly sensitive to negative responses – or responses from other people that attempt to pull them into the everyday reality that those of us without this disease experience.

At one point, my mother began having difficulties with choosing what to eat from a menu.

"Mom, maybe you would like the chicken salad, or would you prefer the Reuben sandwich?" I offer. I see confusion on her face as she says, "Yes, I'll have that. But don't mix in the dessert. I want it in my purse."

"Do you think you'll have room in your purse for that big piece of pie?" I ask.

"I always have room" Mom says as she looks up with a twinkle in her eye, as her mouth starts to widen into a laugh.

Another time, I walk into the living room, approaching my parents' two recliner chairs from behind. My mom is seated in her chair, but there is something strange on top of her head. I come around to face her. My breath catches, and then I break out into a big smile and laugh as I ask, "Mom, what have got on your head?"

"Hats, can't you see?" she says with obvious chagrin, and a bit of huffiness, as anyone would be able to see the obvious, and as if to say, "What's wrong with you?"

In fact, she has a stack of hats on her head, all different colors, blending nicely with her very colorful top. I burst into laughter, and my mother joins in this light moment with me, with a big laugh and a huge smile when I photograph her with her special head gear. This event was one of many times during my mother's Alzheimer's years in which I was able to get her to laugh simultaneously with me. In dealing with people with Alzheimer's, it is critical to not laugh AT them but to laugh WITH them. As stated earlier, all of their emotions and sensitivities are intact, and they know when they are being condescended to or criticized.

In that incident, I also interpreted the stack of hats as a symbol of what my mother was going through – layers of hats, and slowly losing her mind, one layer at a time. My aunt, Joan Yates, later told me another piece of family history that neither I nor my siblings had ever heard and that may have also had some connection to my mother's behavior. According to Aunt Joan, when my mother's older sister Helen was a teenager, (perhaps fifteen or sixteen), she left the family ranch in Wyoming where she had been sent to live with my mother and their brother, Howard, sometime after their early abandonment by my grandmother. Helen went back to Philadelphia to live with their mother, Frieda. However, as an adult, Helen told aunt Joan that she had to eventually leave her mother in order to save her own life. Frieda, was literally not feeding her. And Frieda took the money for food and bought hats! This family story becomes even more fascinating with the apparent connection to my mother's love of hats.

As for Helen, she found a Catholic church where the nuns took her in and cared for her. My aunt Helen told Joan, "I would have died if the Catholic nuns had not taken me in." This experience also explains my aunt Helen's conversion to Catholicism later in life, and her attempts to get my mother to do the same. My mother would have nothing to do with that effort. She was not interested in forgiving Frieda, as her sister Helen had done, and certainly had no interest in converting from her Episcopalian faith to Catholicism.

When their mother, Frieda, died in 1963, my mother did not shed a tear. Her mother had been eliminated from her life and her consciousness many years before. This story from aunt Joan points to the clear mental health issues exhibited by my grandmother, of narcissism and such self-centeredness to the point where she would endanger her own child's life by not even feeding Helen. After hearing this story, I realized that my grandmother's self-centeredness was what my mother had spoken of to me when I was a young child.

Trying to understand how my grandmother could have acted as she did, I went into meditation one day and asked Frieda to tell me why she did not provide food for her daughter, Helen, her first born child. Here is how she responded:

*"I felt overwhelmed. I felt she was taking from me. I felt that I had to protect everything I had worked hard to achieve. I felt there wasn't enough for all of us. There were dark forces that made me feel outside of myself, that made me pull into myself. At times, I didn't understand what was happening but I knew I had to protect myself. The world began to feel unsafe to me. I felt I had disappointed my father because of the man I had married and also because the marriage failed. I couldn't bear to see my family and have them judge me. I knew I had failed in their eyes and I could not face it."*

Later, I also wanted to understand how my mother, Ada, could erase Frieda from her life. As I focused on inwardly hearing my mother's voice, I found it quite disturbing to feel into the darkness of her Alzheimer's disease, as she related these insights to me:

*"I wanted to put my mother out of my mind, and out of my life, as if she never existed. And yet, you cannot erase the truth and the facts. I am grateful that I was raised with so much love from Aunt Bessie, (her father's sister) and grateful that she taught me so many lessons in life. I tried to practice the love that Aunt*

*Bessie taught me, and knew that holding resentment and hatred in my heart would only harm me. I felt I had to be careful when answering questions about my mother, at least to a limited extent. I know a child's curiosity, but it was too painful for me to speak much about my mother and my early beginnings.*

*Yes, the Alzheimer's connects to my erasing part of my early experiences. No accident that my mind began to disappear as I had erased part of it early on. As I look back, that period of my life was also an attempt to experience the total love and care that that I missed from my mother. I became like a small child who needed constant looking after. But more than that, it was a path to experiencing the cocoon of love and care that I missed from my mother. It allowed me to be held and loved like a small child. I have few memories of receiving that from my mother. I now know she was incapable of giving me that. She didn't get it from her mother. She was the eldest in her family and was expected to be mature and responsible, and to care for her younger siblings. A tall order for a young girl."*

# CHAPTER 5

# A Portrait of my Mother Before Alzheimer's

My mother was a study in perfection, as the perfectionist in her aimed to accomplish everything at a very high level. To me, she seemed a living garden of every imaginable flower, every color of the rainbow. Her soul was the sweetest scent of gardenias that she grew outside the front door. She was the glory of tall iris that she had in the backyard for a short time. She taught me about nature and to appreciate its mysteries and to revel in its beauty. When a fresh blanket of snow covered the morning ground and its bright reflection seeped under the bedroom curtains, no one was more excited about the prospect of school being closed for the day than my mother, so that her children could be home with her to play in the snow. And no one more enjoyed a walk out in its biting crispness.

My mother was a professional walker. She could walk the pants off anyone, even half her age. Probably most of all, my mother loved the ocean, walking the beach and looking for seashells. She could hardly contain herself in anticipation of the midnight grunion run on the beach in San Diego where we would vacation. Millions of tiny female silver grunion fish wash up on the beach at very high tide to lay their eggs. The male fish then wrap themselves around the females to deposit their sperm. For ten days the grunion eggs remain hidden in the sand before hatching and washing out to sea at the next set of high tides. My mother would squeal with delight at all the millions of sparkling, slithering tiny silver fish all over the beach.

From cowgirl to beach girl, my mother simply loved nature. And she was a sharpshooter. As a young woman in 1939, she was the intercollegiate Small Bore National Rifle Champion. The trophy for that accomplishment is still in our family.

My mother was also a professional newspaper clipper. She made it her job to keep everyone around her informed of important events, developments and special news items tailored for each person's interests. She had a separate file for each person, stuffed with clippings she would collect and mail. My mother was also a professional organizer. Everything had a place and everything was usually in its place. My mother worked as a secretary in the English Department at Chico State, the college in Chico, twelve miles from Paradise, the town that made national news when it was decimated by wildfire in 2018. We used to say that she ran the whole department, probably not much of an exaggeration.

And it was she alone who had organized a houseful of belongings when our family of five moved to Japan in 1953 from Cheyenne, Wyoming, including three small children and the piano too! My father was in the Air Force, part of the troops assigned to rebuild Japan after the war. We lived in a friendly Japanese neighborhood in Nagoya, in a typical Japanese house, that came with a Japanese maid. However, our stay only lasted about four months, as the Air Force decided they did not need so many men and sent hundreds of them home, including my father. We moved first to Menlo Park, California, and my father finished his M.A. degree in Education Administration at Stanford. He was then offered a position as the principal of the elementary school in Paradise, California, and we moved there in 1954 when I was five years old. I grew up in Paradise and left after graduating from high school to attend the University of California, Berkeley.

After retiring from Chico State, my mother jumped into many activities, several of which she had been active in for years: League of Women Voters, Children's Home Society, Community Concerts Association, Paradise Symphony Association, local politics and community activities. She would spend hours on the phone enrolling people into various organizations and political campaigns, and persuading them of the importance of their active participation in community affairs. As my father was an educator, and she shared his passion for learning, my mother spent a great deal of time talking to Paradise residents about the importance of supporting education and electing school board members who would represent the best educational opportunities for local students. And my mother read voraciously. She belonged to several book clubs and new books were always arriving at the house, as well as several magazine subscriptions such as *Harper's, New Republic, The Nation,* and *National Geographic.* When I was younger, *Life* magazine was a staple in our house. I will never forget the 1963 spread on President Kennedy's assassination in that large magazine.

My mother also loved to cook. She became a reformed practitioner of the cook-it-to-death 1950's, totally transformed by Julia Child's revolution that brought French culinary techniques to Americans. Cooking is one of the places where her creativity shined. She also loved flowers and gardens, but in my years of growing up at home, my overcontrolling father left her limited space to grow the flowers she wanted. Nevertheless, my mother did plant many flowers that she enjoyed, perhaps as her way of standing up to my father and staking out her space. She did not simply give in to him, and her flowers made a statement about what was important to her. My father had established himself as the master gardener. He had perhaps 600 rhododendrons, azaleas and camellias in the front and backyards. In addition to dozens of tall oak, pine and manzanita trees, my father also planted about twenty giant coastal redwood seedlings, of which about ten grew to maturity. Our yard was quite impressive, especially in the spring when everything bloomed at once. The front and backyards were a mass of color that was once featured in *Sunset* Magazine. Every year, people would drive from miles away to come see the spectacular display.

These memories make me think about the parts of my parent's relationship that were dysfunctional, and how my mother had shut down aspects of herself to survive with my father. She had also lived through my father's emotional abuse of my brother, who was eight years older than me. That experience would have been another way in which my mother closed her heart. As I stated earlier, it is my belief that her closed heart was a contributing factor in her Alzheimer's, as well as the depression she struggled with after I, her last child, had left home for college. My mother did argue a lot with my father, and did stand up to him. However, I think she knew how to pick her battles. Rather than arguing with my father about finances or about making a donation to one of her favorite charities, she would simply write a check to the charitable organization and not tell my father. Besides, she managed the money anyway. My mother once attempted to improve their marriage by going to a family therapist. Since my father refused to go, however, the therapist told her he could not help them unless my father was willing to come in for therapy too.

This brilliant woman, who graduated Magna Cum Laude in Mathematics at age nineteen from the University of Wyoming in Laramie, would have made a substantial mark of her own in some way had she lived in another era than the 1950s. But in her later years during the 1990s, she was on a downhill slide. And my whole family couldn't and didn't want to see it, including me…at least in the beginning.

As it turns out, our family was typical – just like many others who did not know how to handle this disease. We all wanted to hold on to the woman we loved…the woman we knew before Alzheimer's.

# CHAPTER 6

# The Bottom Drops Out

By late 1995 – five years after getting that first glimmer of my mother's condition when Jim and I were in Tahiti – my mother's Alzheimer's had progressed to the point where she was like a small child who could not be left alone. As she continued to decline, I knew a crisis was inevitable. Intuitively, I knew that it was time to put her in some type of out of home placement, but my father could not face this next step. While I felt the storm clouds were bound to break sooner or later, I could not have known in advance just what form the disaster would take. It wasn't long, though, before I found out.

One stormy night in February 1996, I received a phone call very early in the morning from Midge, the neighbor who lived across the street from my parents in Paradise. "Marilyn, you've got to get up here," she frantically told me. "There's been a fire at your house. Your mom is staying with Martha, (an elderly next-door neighbor), and your dad is in the hospital with third degree burns."

I was shocked, and again fearful for my parents' safety. I suppressed my fears and worry, and pushed down the tears that I couldn't let fall in that moment. In short order, I was on the road, driving the three hours from the Bay Area to Paradise.

When I arrived at Martha's house, my mother was awake and dressed, sitting calmly with Martha having tea and breakfast. She smiled at me, and I hugged her. I was relieved to see my mother was well cared for, and thanked Martha for taking her in.

Once I knew Mom was settled, I went next door to inspect the house. I gasped at what confronted me, and felt shock waves going through my body. The fire had totally gutted the garage and the two cars that had been parked inside, which were now only twisted shells of metal. It had destroyed part of my parent's bedroom next to the garage and then raged across the long, narrow back porch leading from the garage to the kitchen. While that was bad enough, there was even more extensive damage caused by smoke throughout the house.

I would have expected that my mother had caused the fire, but no, it was my father. For years they had heated their house with a fireplace insert, which my father stoked from the huge woodpile in the backyard. For years he had carefully tended the fireplace, removing the ashes when they had built up. He used to place those ashes in a big incinerator in the backyard. But this time, after allowing the ashes to cool in a pail on the back porch for perhaps two days, he had then emptied then into the garbage can in the garage. Why this change in routine, I will never know. The ashes were not sufficiently cooled. The garage was closed with two cars in it, both with full tanks of gas. The heat from the ashes in that closed environment sparked the fire and then the gas tanks exploded and fueled its spread.

Midge's husband, Ed, a retired fireman, gave me a detailed description of what had happened. He knew my parent's routine and kept a close eye on them. On this winter afternoon, Ed heard popping noises and recognized the sounds of fire, and immediately swung into action. Flagging down a passing motorist who also turned out to be another retired fireman, (what are the chances of that!), they ran to my parents' house. Ed knew that at this time of day, my parents would be napping in their recliner chairs in the living room. He first tried the front door, but it was locked. He and the second fireman raced around to the back kitchen door, and luckily, it was unlocked. As Ed had thought, my parents were indeed both asleep in their chairs. Knowing that my mother would not be able to follow instructions, Ed yelled, "Al, get that front door open! We've got to get Ada out!" With the door unlocked, he and the second fireman carried my mother to Martha's house next door and deposited her there before going back to the burning house.

My father was not one to avoid danger. In fact, he had a history of flirting with danger and in this case, he went toward it. Rather than getting away from the fire as fast as possible, he opened the back kitchen door to go investigate. The kitchen door faced the garage across a long narrow cement porch.

That action drew the flames toward him. Luckily, he had his eyeglasses on. As the flames rushed toward him, he instinctively put his hands over his eyes and consequently suffered third degree burns on the top of his head and the backs of his hands. That action landed him in the hospital where he underwent painful skin graft surgery.

After the fire, I had to remain in Paradise for three weeks, staying with Martha who had taken in my mother. Martha was so gracious and welcoming, and gave her bed to my mother. She took up residence in the second bedroom and I set myself up in the upstairs attic bedroom. From my first day there, I was constantly in motion or on the phone, making arrangements with house and car insurance agents, smoke cleaning services, utility line workers, and building contractors. The phone at Martha's house rang constantly, as did the front doorbell. You would think that all this activity was a major intrusion on an elderly woman accustomed to quietly living alone. Martha, however, seemed to be lit up with my activities and the bustle in the house.

I had to balance all these goings-on while attending to my mother's needs and not leaving her alone with Martha, who had agreed to watch my mother for short periods of time – usually around two hours. I started searching for a facility where I could place my mother, as soon as possible. I did not discuss this with her, as she had long since lost the ability to follow such a conversation and make decisions, much less participate in the search. My mother seemed to also enjoy this new residence with Martha, as she was finally out from under my father's control.

In his needy state, my father frequently called me from the hospital. "When are you coming to see me?" he asks. "How is mother?"

He inquired about the house. I'm not sure about what he knew in terms of the extent of the destruction, so I evaded his questions a bit. His phone calls felt demanding.

I also received return calls from board and care homes I was looking into for my mother. I was so busy I had no time to process the reality of the next stage of life for my parents, the heart wrenching realization that I needed to place my mother in a safe place, and that would mean the separation of my parents. Only when I finally fell into bed in exhaustion each night, did I allow reality to set in. A few tears made their way down my cheeks. My heart ached.

When things finally calmed down a little, Mom and I make the trip to Chico to visit Dad in the hospital. We enter the front door of Enloe Hospital. I am hit with the hospital smell of strong disinfectant, covered over with some type of overpowering perfume odor. Before finding our way to my dad's room, it occurs to me that making a bathroom stop would be a good idea for both my mother and me. We enter the women's restroom. My mom goes into the last stall, I use the one next to her. As I finish up washing my hands, I say to my mom, "I'll wait for you outside."

"OK!" I hear her chirpy voice say. Outside, I'm waiting and people watching. A little girl, about four years old, is being pulled along by a woman who says to her, "Let's hurry, honey. Sissy is waiting for us." The mom looks stressed, the little girl strains at being pulled along faster than she can keep up. An older man with white hair, stooped shoulders and a cane, shuffles slowly and carefully as he walks along the carpeted floor. I meet his eye briefly, and see the tiredness, and yet the resolve in his gaze.

I suddenly realize several minutes have gone by and my mother has not emerged from the restroom. I re-enter the restroom to check on her.

"*Mom, are you alright?*"

"*Yup.*"

I walk to the last stall to check on her progress and open the door. My mother is standing there, fully clothed, but there is one unique change to her appearance. She is now wearing the paper seat cover over her head, and it's placed neatly around her neck! I am so shocked and bemused that I barely manage to say, "Here, let me help you." I remove the new head gear from around her neck and throw it away.

"*Do you still need to go?*"

"*Nope.*"

Before we leave the restroom, I make sure she has everything in place. I quickly go out the door and don't know whether to laugh or cry as I explode into simultaneous laughter and tears.

My mother exits the restroom and we make our way upstairs to my father's hospital room. When we enter his room, his face lights up upon seeing us.

"Here you are!" he exclaims, clearly excited to see both of us. I am shocked to see his legs and forehead all bandaged up, having temporarily blocked out of my mind the cause of his being here in the hospital and suffering through third degree burns.

My mom seems a little confused as to why he is here, and hesitantly approaches his bed.

"Hi doll! I'm so happy to see you!" my father exclaims. She says nothing, and has a somewhat empty look on her face. My father takes my mother's hand in his and speaks softly to her. "How is my sweetheart?" My father and I chat a bit about what's happening with the house, and I assure him that everything is getting handled. He seems to relax as he realizes that I've got the house situation under control. He keeps gazing at my mother with an adoring, yet concerned look on his face. She still seems disoriented and puzzled as to why he is here in the hospital. We soon leave my father, with assurances that he is healing well and looks strong.

In the middle of all the overwhelm of handling everything with the burned house, looking for a care home for my mother and making sure her needs were met, and fielding phone calls from my father in the hospital, I am feeling exhausted and emotionally pushed to my limit. Then one day I receive a phone call from the hospital to inform me that my father is going to be discharged. No one had consulted with me, and no discharge nurse had let me know of the plans to release him from the hospital. No one had asked about the housing situation for my father. I am completely flummoxed, caught off guard and angry. I am so overwhelmed and not thinking straight. Who had made this decision? Why hadn't I been consulted about this in advance? Well, I thought, they must think he's ready for discharge. I drive to Chico the next day to pick him up and bring him back to Martha's house in Paradise. We put him in the bedroom with my mother and I move from the attic bedroom to the second bedroom, next to my parents. Martha moves to the couch in the living room.

This release of my father turns out to be the most disastrous and outrageous move on the part of the hospital. My father still has leaking wounds on his legs where the skin had been peeled off for grafts. He is not steady on his feet. And the worst part is his incontinence and need for frequent trips to the bathroom. I am up about every two hours throughout the night assisting my father to the bathroom. This was the point at which all boundaries and privacy between father and daughter went out the window. Not only am I having to assist him in getting to the toilet, I also have to assist him with getting his pants down and onto the toilet. I had never performed such a task with anyone, much less my father. Up until this time, both my parents were dealing with incontinence but had managed with washable, reusable large diaper briefs.

By the morning, I am frazzled, overwhelmed and exhausted. I phone the hospital and speak to a nurse in charge. "My father was released prematurely from your hospital, without consultation with me, his daughter. He is in no way prepared to be home, and belongs in the hospital. His wounds are leaking, he's in pain, and unable to care for himself. He is incontinent and requires assistance with toileting. I am his daughter, not a nurse." She informs me that his daughter *had* given permission for him to be released. "What???? What are you talking about?? I AM the daughter, and I never gave permission for him to be discharged!!" She replied, "I'm sorry, there is nothing I can do. He has been released."

I am completely undone. I then call my close childhood friend Patty, a nurse, the daughter of my parents' best friends, Evelyn and Bill. She happened to be in Paradise that weekend visiting her dad. I break down crying on the phone, telling Patty that I cannot cope with this any longer. To my huge relief, she says, "I'll be right over." It was no more than twenty minutes later when Patty showed up. I melt in tears into her arms. She looked at my dad's leg wounds and agreed that he still belonged in the hospital. Patty called the hospital and explained the situation, but they were unwilling to take my father back.

Perhaps a year or two later, I learned from a sister of Patty's who had contacts inside the hospital where my father had been a patient, that it had been my sister calling from Germany who gave permission for my dad to be released from the hospital. She and I were estranged, and she had not been a part of all the decision making regarding my parents' situation. So, thanks to my sister's ill-informed action, my father would be leaving the hospital and going to a house that was far from equipped for his homecoming.

◆

A few days later came one of the most difficult parts of this whole journey. I had checked out some facilities for my mother and had selected a board and care facility in Chico that had a cozy home-like setting with only about six residents. The owner seemed attentive and caring. Her home was clean and inviting, there was no smell of urine or disinfectant, and the residents appeared to be well taken care of. I packed up some of my mother's belongings and loaded my mother into the car. I did not tell her where we were going or what was happening, as she would not have understood. Alzheimer's patients live in the moment, and do not have the ability to follow a concept from point A to point B. What is most prominent for them are their emotions.

As far as my own emotions, I was barely keeping them in check as we traveled the twelve miles down the hill to Chico. Arriving at the care home, we were warmly greeted by the owner, a middle-aged woman who communicated openness and earthiness. "Welcome! Come on in!", she said. She showed us into the small bedroom that would be my mother's room. It had a single bed, a small dresser, a gingham covered overstuffed chair, and windows with curtains that let in soft light. I never even looked out the window to see what was there. I set my mother's belongings down, and then sat on the edge of the bed with her. Mustering up my courage, and with a heavy heart, I said to her, "This is going to be your new home. You need more help and care than Dad is able to give you. They will take good care of you here and you will be safe. I will come to visit you and bring Dad to visit when he is able to come."

I remember the faraway look in her eyes, and yet there was also a flicker of recognition, of knowing she would never return home, that life had changed dramatically and suddenly. Her fingers fumbled with each other, knit together, then searched for a new comfortable place to rest, as if seeking a new home in which to live. She said nothing, but I could see sadness in her eyes. Tears streamed down my cheeks. After a few final words with the owner, telling her that I would check in with her in a couple days, I went back out to my car. It was then that I burst into tears. I knew this was the right thing, but I felt my heart tearing apart, the grief of this relentless downward spiral with no hope for recovery or reversal. I knew it was the first step in my mother's final descent, but I had no idea how long that would take and where it would lead.

Driving back to Paradise, I was flooded with memories of the innumerable trips up and down that road in better times with my mother – the fun shopping trips to Chico for new clothes for both of us, the ice cream parlor where we indulged in our favorites, chocolate mint chip of course, the outings to restaurants such as Gino's, our favorite Italian restaurant, the visits to longtime friends in Chico. I was also reminded of my mother's horticultural training with me, naming the Scotch broom and redbud plants that we passed as we traveled back home. We would marvel at all the beautiful trees in full leaf and bloom, as well as the clarity of the air in the canyon beside the road that led back to Paradise. So many years, so many memories!

A couple days later, I drove down to visit my mother in Chico. I was relieved and happy to find that she was adapting well to her new home. When I walked in the front door, she was seated in the living room recliner chair. Her smile and the contented look on her face communicated all I needed to know. She seemed to have settled in and was beginning to make new friends.

Perhaps a week later, I made another visit to my mom. This time, it was clear that she had indeed made some new friends. In fact, her flirtatiousness again blossomed in this new setting. My mother had taken a liking to another resident, Joe, a tall, lanky man whose easy drawl and manner welcomed all in his presence. Joe was an avid reader, much like my mother. And he looked like a cowboy, another common thread between he and my mother who'd spent her childhood years on the ranch in Wyoming. However, Joe was mentally competent and was in this care setting because of physical limitations. For what other reasons, I did not know.

The staff told me during this visit about a very funny incident involving Joe and my mother. Joe often sat in his bedroom reading, which was next to my mother's room. One day, as he was reading, my mother suddenly appeared at his open door, padded over to his bed, and proceeded to climb into it! "Ada, what are you doing?" Joe blurted out. "You're going to get me in trouble!" She turned to him, put an index finger to her lips, and said, "Shhhhh" and snuggled further under the covers. Joe was astonished, but what could he do? The staff related this incident to me with giggles and we had tears running down our cheeks from our shared laughter. It was, perhaps, as entertaining for them as it was for me. I was finally able to relax, knowing that my mother was apparently adjusting quite well.

On another visit, I heard about the day when a staff member went into my mother's room and found her sitting in her chair, stark naked. She had a book in her hands. The staff member said to her, "Ada, what are you doing?" She replied, "Reading, can't you see?"

The staff and I cracked up at this! I was so grateful to have my mother in a home where she felt free and safe to express herself, and to know that the staff would respond with humor and acceptance, not judgment or punitive measures.

Because of the extensive smoke cleaning of every single item and surface in my parents' house and the rebuilding of the house itself – including installation of central heating for the first time ever – my father was not able to return to the house for a month after he stabilized from his release from the hospital. Synchronistically, my friend Patty's father, Bill, who was my father's close friend, had lost his wife just before the fire at my parents' house. So they were both dealing with the loss of their wives, and sharing their grief, though my mother was still in this world. It was the perfect short-term resolution to my father having no home to return to after the fire, and Bill rattling around in his enormous house by himself. They truly embodied the male characters from movies like "The Odd Couple", or "Grumpy Old Men", which was quite entertaining from the outside. Each of them complained about the other to their daughters. My father would say, "He never washes the dishes! Just lets them pile up!" Bill would complain, "Al just sits around all day, doing nothing."

When it was time to return to his house, my father started talking about taking my mother back to our family home. I had to have a conversation with him about the importance of leaving her in the care home in Chico. I had to reframe the conversation so that my father could take it in, as his fierce loyalty to my mother was so apparent. And of course, he had never lived alone in the house without his life partner. I could feel his apprehension. "Dad, you have done a fantastic job of taking care of Mom all these years, but now you deserve a break," I told him. "You need to take care of yourself. You can't continue to carry the weight of taking care of Mom. She's in a good home and well taken care of. And you'll be able to visit her regularly." He had come to rely on me for major decisions, and in hindsight, I think he needed my permission to let go and make this difficult move, one that he never would have made on his own. In the end, he was so happy to move back to his own home, which was essentially brand new, and to be able to turn on the heat or cooling air by simply flicking a switch. That in itself was an enormous freedom for him.

My mother remained in the care home for seven months, and then that plateau ended, and she declined further. Her Alzheimer's disease had been a journey of long plateaus before dropping to the next lower level. At this point, it was time to move her from the board and care home and into a full-fledged nursing home in Chico, where she remained for two years before her passing. The nursing home I chose was clean and fairly new, did not smell of urine or unpleasant odors, the staff seemed attentive and caring and the food was at least passable. And they did not have recorded incidents of complaints. In choosing a nursing home, or any care home, researching complaints is a critical part of the process of selection. You must ask about incidents, and the facility must show them to you.

By this time, my mother had become incontinent, non-verbal and unable to feed herself. But her basic sweet personality still lit up the room when my mother was "present" that is, when she was aware in the current moment, and not lost in the fog of Alzheimer's. In this facility, the staff competed to take care of her.

As it turns out, a young woman aide was assigned as my mother's primary caretaker. Sarah was a jewel. She went far beyond the call of duty in caring for my mother – as if my mom was her own mother. In fact, what I witnessed was a psychological/emotional transference to my mother that transcended the patient/caregiver relationship. Sarah would bring in her own Calgon bath oil beads, put my mother in a bathtub laced with the beads, and light a candle. She would then give my mother a neck and shoulder massage. She would bring in her three-year old daughter who loved to sit on my mother's bed while my mother delightedly played with her and Sarah read stories.

The most touching display of love and care was when Sarah told me that she would get into my mother's bed with her when she could tell that my mother was scared, or terrified. I was blown away at the level of care that went so far beyond what one would expect. There truly are miracle workers in these settings. When my mother did pass, Sarah had to take some time off her job to recover. My mother had been her first patient to die.

For the two years that my mother was at the nursing home, my father would drive from Paradise to Chico every day to feed my mom and visit. He became a fixture on her ward, and the staff enjoyed having someone mentally competent and intelligent with whom they could converse. The staff became my father's surrogate family. "We love having him here," they would tell me. "He's so interesting."

About a year before my mother's passing, my father's prostate cancer returned and had spread throughout his body. Eventually he was hospitalized at the same facility in which my mother resided, but in a different ward. When his insurance stopped the coverage in that ward, he told me he was going to transfer to my mother's ward. I said to him, "But Dad, that whole ward is for Alzheimer's and brain-impaired patients." I was concerned about his going to that ward as he was mentally competent. He replied, "No, you don't understand. I've been going there every day for two years to see Mom. The staff are like my family." My father was placed in a separate room a few doors down the hallway from my mom. They were together again at last, and of course were able to be with each other every day.

I continued to make frequent trips to Chico to visit both my parents and check on my mother's status. She continued to deteriorate, and at this stage, she was in and out of being present in her body. She had been non-verbal for quite a long time, but her eyes often communicated love and connection. Other times, her eyes were vacant and she seemed lost in another world. Sometimes she would know who I was, sometimes not. What I did not know, and was fearful about, was how long she would last and whether she would slide into the most difficult advanced stage of Alzheimer's where even the physical autonomic system begins to shut down. I dreaded the possibility of her developing an inability to swallow.

As it turned out, my father died ten months before my mother, in November 1997. I spoke with him on the phone on a Friday afternoon. He said, "I'm in so much pain, I've been having thoughts of dying." My father had never spoken this way, and throughout his life and every physical ordeal, he was always determined and had a very high tolerance for pain. For him to speak of dying was, I knew, the beginning of the end. I threw some belongings together and left for Chico soon after that conversation.

Upon arriving at the nursing home, I entered my father's room to find him in bed, the pain etched on his face. After he repeated that he had been having thoughts of dying, I immediately launched into the most important conversation I had ever had with him. "Dad, when you are ready to go, that decision is completely up to you," I told him. "We are all fine, Mom is taken care of, I'm doing well, Louise (my sister) is fine. It's okay to let go." I could immediately see the relief on his face. And we cried together.

I knew that my father's fierce loyalty to family and love for all of us, was the driving force in his thinking. In his mind, he was the provider and the one looking over everyone, and he worried about my mother and sister in particular.

The next few days with him after that deep conversation were precious, as I brought him special food requests, and had lighter conversations about shared memories. I also witnessed an amazing transformation into what I have to call a state of radiance, with a light and peace emanating from within my father that I had never seen in anyone. He was not nor had he ever been religious or spiritual. But this transformation was palpable. Two days later he was gone. I knew he had reached a true place of peace.

Shortly after his passing, as my mother didn't see my father making his way to her room, speaking softly to her, or feeding her, I realized that she knew he was gone. She had been non-verbal for some time, but I could feel an emptiness in her presence that had not been there before my father's death.

# CHAPTER 7

# Saying Goodbye to my Mother

In July 1998, I set out on a solo two-week road trip I had wanted to make for a long time. When I was a child, my family had gone on many vacations to Wyoming, to visit family and friends in Cheyenne, where I was born. We'd also go to the ranch about two hours outside of Cheyenne, where my mother grew up. I envisioned this trip as something of a "vision quest" for me. I wanted to go deep within myself, to be with my heart and listen for messages or guidance. I wanted to connect with and feel the presence of the Divine. I also wanted to connect with ancestors and to be open to receiving messages. I could not have known the divine portent this trip would turn out to be.

I love driving, I love travel, and I loved retracing the roads that my family had driven on in years past. I was well stocked with books on tape and music cassettes. As this was just the beginning of the ubiquitous cell phone, I did not own such a device. I borrowed a friend's bulky portable phone and felt safer having it on my solo adventure. This was also a time when making lodging reservations ahead of time was unnecessary. I easily found adequate motels in which to stay along the way.

My first destination was Saratoga, Wyoming, where my uncle Howard, my mother's brother, and his wife, Vernice, lived. We spent a lovely four days together at their lake-side home, in which I learned much about my grandmother, Frieda. When Howard was in his mid-twenties, he had returned to Philadelphia to live with his mother for about a year. He told me of her self-absorption and narcissism.

After that year, a family friend of Frieda's told Howard, "You will never get what you're looking for from your mother. You just need to leave." Obviously, he was seeking the love and care that he had never received from her. He left, and never looked back or had contact with his mother again.

From Saratoga, my next stop was Cheyenne, my birthplace. However, since we had moved from Cheyenne when I was two years old, I had no memories of it. The meaning it had for me was the many fun vacations staying at uncle Howard's big multi-level house, a house that seemed magical to me with its many staircases, laundry chute, and a separate family TV room. Another magical and fun thing was riding around town with uncle Howard in his private black hearse, a vehicle which he had purchased to use as an everyday car. Howard definitely had a sense of humor, albeit very dry.

I didn't go to that house on this trip, however. Instead, I stayed with my mother's closest friend from college, Muriel, and her husband, Gene. They took me in like their own daughter, wined and dined me and shared stories with me of their friendship over the years with my mother. With Muriel's warmth and open heart, as well as her brilliance, I could see why she and my mother had remained friends all these years since college. I visited other old friends of my mother's in Cheyenne. Everyone was glad to get an update on my mother but all were sad to learn of her advancing Alzheimer's, and my father's passing.

From Cheyenne, I drove out to the ranch near La Grange where my mother grew up. Bumping my way down the dirt and gravel road, and clattering over the cattleguards, I felt the same excitement I had experienced during childhood as I approached the ranch. The low, dark yellow hills rising in the distance, the scrub brush all round, fields of yellow dead grass, and sparse vegetation brought memories flooding back to me of long horse rides over the countryside, playing in the nearby creek, and marveling at the collection of farm animals which included cows, pigs and horses. My car tires crunched over the gravel driveway, and as I jumped out of the car, I was suddenly eight or ten years old again. My nostrils were filled with barnyard smells and old house scents, the memory of newly mowed hay in the distance. I was warmly greeted by my two cousins, Cheri and Bob. I hadn't been to the ranch for perhaps thirty-five years. The house had definitely aged, but still had the familiar odor of unhomogenized, unpasteurized milk, and old furniture. Or perhaps, I was lost in my early memories of what had been to me, another magical childhood experience. There were no more cows and horses, but as I stood out in the yard, I could sense the horse's strong withers beneath me, and the breeze brushing my face as we galloped over the land. I felt my mother's presence, and imagined her smiling from ear to ear as she returned to her childhood home in spirit.

What I did not realize until after I had returned from this trip, was that I had been unconsciously preparing my mother for making her transition from this earth plane. I was completing the circuit for her, touching base with all the special people and places of her younger life, taking the journey for her so that she could make her passing. No wonder she felt so present for me on that trip!

From Wyoming, I drove down through Colorado. This was the state where my father had grown up. He had gone to college at Colorado State University in Fort Collins, and I went there to visit his alma mater. I stopped at a store and bought a sandwich for lunch, then parked near the campus and walked onto a very large expanse of beautifully kept lawn, bordered on two sides by large buildings. I sat on the lawn eating my lunch, and wondered to myself where Dad's fraternity was. I then heard an inward voice speak to me, "Turn around. It's right behind you." I had to get up to go look at the beautiful wood and stone building behind me, and was astonished to see that it was in fact, my father's fraternity house!

As I walked back to the spot where I had been eating my lunch, I again received an inner prompting, "Go over to that building on the right. You will hear some beautiful music coming from there." Having been already guided by this voice to the fraternity, I had to follow through and investigate. I walked up a flight of stairs, and was almost bowled over by the sounds of a small live orchestra playing the most beautiful music somewhere in the building, though I couldn't see where it was coming from.

My father was clearly guiding me during this stage of the journey. Music had been a huge part of my parents' lives and classical music was always playing on the radio in our house, including Saturday broadcasts of opera, (to the huge consternation of my teenage ears as I tried to sleep late!). My parents, my sister and I also frequently attended live concerts of classical artists.

These experiences of my mom and dad's origins, their young lives and young adult friendships gave me a much fuller portrait of them as people, not just my parents. When I set out on this trip, I did not realize that it would be a journey of completion for my father, who had passed eight months earlier. What was even more astonishing and unpredictable to me was completing the journey for my mother. Little did I know at the time that I'd only have one more month with her.

My sister, Louise, had returned from Germany several months before and eventually moved back to our childhood home a few months before my mother's passing. When it was clear that my mother was near the end of her life, my sister and I organically and spontaneously formed a unified team to care for my mother in her last four days. Despite our long-standing conflicts and difficult relationship, we were able to put that all aside and be there totally for my mother, focused only on helping to make her passing as peaceful and easy as possible. I was grateful for and amazed at our teamwork – even more so today, after I learned of her role in the premature release of my father from the hospital back in 1996. We had a common purpose in caring for Mom that transcended the many tensions and arguments we had had over the years. We read poetry to her, we massaged and caressed her, we talked to her about what a good mother she had been, and we mostly stayed close with her to accompany her on this final journey. Occasionally, she would sit bolt upright in bed, as if she had seen a vision, or perhaps angels. At times she was clearly fearful, and at other times she appeared to be sleeping peacefully.

After two days of being with my mother continuously, the nurses offered to clear out the community common room for us. I was blown away by this generous offer, and so grateful. They moved all the residents out of that room, which had a television for them to watch. They moved my mother's bed into that room and set up two extra beds for my sister and me. We had the entire large room entirely to ourselves for two days.

My sister and I said, "We've got to find music for her since it was such an important part of her life." We turned on the TV. Miraculously, we found the Arts and Culture channel, with non-stop, continuous music of live performances of classical music, ballet, symphonies, solo singers, small chamber orchestras and more, uninterrupted by ads or anything. So many of my mother's favorite, beloved pieces emanated from the television, Chopin concertos, Debussy's "Clair De Lune", and Ravel's "Bolero". When Tchaikovsky's "Swan Lake" came on, my mother suddenly came to life and sat straight up, her eyes bright and riveted on the TV.

Her final passing was peaceful, with my sister reading to her the well-known passage from the Bible, Psalm 23, "Yea, though I walk through the valley of the shadow of death, I will fear no evil: for thou art with me."

On September 22, 1998, my mother passed away.

I felt again, as I had felt with my father's passing, that I had been given a gift, the gift of bearing witness to a beautiful life, and being present with the beautiful, though painful, passing through the gate to whatever lies beyond. I felt transformed.

# CHAPTER 8

# Healing My Own Closed Heart

My mother's death in 1998 did not end our intimate connection. While it didn't always register consciously, I could still somewhat sense her presence as we went through all of the steps involved in closing up my parent's estate and selling the family home. After all the stresses that many Alzheimer's caregivers experience, I had to decompress for a while and find my way back to a more balanced way of living.

The year after my mother's death was another difficult chapter of dealing with my siblings, since I was the executor of my family's affairs. I was responsible for clearing out the house and preparing it for sale. I had hoped to avoid the conflicts that many people go through with siblings when a parent's death brings up all the unresolved family dynamics, but that was not the card I drew. It was a year of my learning to set boundaries and to speak the truth, even when my siblings didn't like what

I was saying or doing, and to know that I was doing the best job I could under difficult circumstances.

Once everything was complete, I then needed to focus on healing myself and my hurting heart. After having provided so much caregiving to my parents, I also needed to unwind from that role and come back to my own career path, as well as attend to my emotional needs. I was grateful for my career and for many supportive friends around me. And I was particularly grateful that a spiritual path opened up before me that provided much healing.

As my divorce became finalized in 2005, I began to immerse myself in the teachings of the Science of Mind through the Oakland Center for Spiritual Living. The Oakland center is part of a larger national organization now called the Centers for Spiritual Living, a spiritual philosophy founded by Ernest Holmes in 1926. These teachings incorporate the ancient wisdom of the world's spiritual traditions including Christian, Jewish, Buddhist, Hindu, Islam and others. I took many courses and workshops, participating in retreats and programs that sparked my deeper relationship with Spirit and the Source of All – all of which expanded my sense of Self and well-being through deep conversations and explorations of life and fulfilling my purpose. I sang in the center's choir for seven years, which included spiritual and gospel music, and had never felt such healing and deep connection with God through music as I did during that experience.

I also had two spiritual teachers who both had a profound effect on me. I first encountered Philip Burley at a daylong workshop in Sacramento, California. Philip is a renowned trance medium, author, and teacher who has been widely known for many years as a trance channel for spiritual master Saint Germain. He has had clairvoyant and clairaudient experiences since childhood. He is also a master teacher of meditation whose students learn to connect with their own inner wisdom, and loving spirit guides. He has had long running radio shows with an international following, as well as ongoing prayer circles by phone, to pray for the healing of the United States. When I connected with Philip, I felt so seen at my deep core, and so at peace with whatever lies beyond this plane of existence. Being seen at that deep level allowed me to connect to my inner gift of intuition and my own spirit guides.

My second deeply impactful spiritual teacher was Charles McCall, now deceased, an ordinary man called from his Snap-On tool business, to give up all attachment to worldly things and to give himself over to guidance from God. Charles was in training for about ten years, sometimes not knowing where his next dime was coming from, but trusting the guidance he was receiving. Ultimately, Charles started direct hands-on healing energy work with individuals, and then added weekend retreats in Southern California. The spiritual work with Charles was deeply transformative and profound. His work was only known by word-of-mouth, but people came from all over the world to participate in his retreats. Charles' work included energy healing, often hands-on, that was extremely powerful. Many modalities of healing were used and taught, all centered on releasing our human self-limitations and self-judgments, and coming to know the divine within ourselves and our connection to the universe.

One of my experiences of healing through this work, occurred around my lifelong fear of being left out, or left behind. During our retreats with Charles, we were transported in vans to restaurants in the area for meals. After breakfast one morning, I went to the restroom, but when I walked out to the parking lot to get into the van in which I had ridden, it was nowhere to be found. I looked all over the parking lot, but no van. It was then that I suddenly realized, I had been left behind! My lifetime fear of being left, had manifested! But instead of panicking, I started laughing hysterically, and continued laughing for several minutes. Because I had established a newfound trust in the universe through this work, I knew I would soon be discovered missing, and that someone would come back for me. I called my friend Sherry, and yes, as soon as my group arrived back at the house where we were all staying, they realized that Marilyn was missing. The van arrived about twenty minutes later. I was still laughing, but definitely relieved.

As part of the many blessings that came through my connection to the Oakland Center for Spiritual Living, I developed a circle of friends, and in January 2018 several of us were part of a tour group to Cuba. The trip was organized by two close friends, Barbara and Marcus. Because of the back story of my mother, and because of my own unconsciousness around my grandmother and her history, it did not even occur to me until we were at the airport waiting to fly out, to tell Marcus the story of my mother and my connection to Cuba.

I explained that my mother and her sister had been born in Cuba – and that my mother had been abandoned at a young age by my grandmother. I also talked about my grandmother's accepting a job in Cuba as an interpreter for Abbott Laboratories. And, I told Marcus about her subsequent marriage to an American cowboy she met in Camaguey. By the time I finished telling this history, Marcus was stunned. "Wow! I've got chills hearing this story!" he exclaimed. "You are definitely meant to go to Cuba."

I am bowled over by the warmth, vibrancy, color and art of Cuba. Javier, our tour guide, is heart centered, very knowledgeable, energetic, and fun. He has an uncanny ability to read people and their needs, and is so expressive and jubilant. We are a joyful group! And that joy is reflected back to us everywhere we go. We are taken for a tour of Havana, riding in several of Cuba's well maintained famous vintage 1950's and '60's American cars. I slide into the slick leather back seat between two friends, and I am suddenly transported to the 1960's. I am sixteen years old, cruising the streets of Chico, California in a convertible '57 Chevy, wedged in the back seat with two girlfriends and another in the front seat between nineteen-year-old driver Bud, and his friend, Steve. The wind is blowing my long blond hair, I am feeling free without a care in the world, and we are looking to party! In Cuba, we wave at people on the sidewalks as we whiz past, and they wave at us, smiles lighting up their faces. The driver gleefully honks the horn as we make our way through the downtown lined with official-looking buildings, next to well-manicured green parks. Javier is riding in our car, and seems to know everyone that we pass as he waves and shouts hello, "Hola Amigo!" He is a fountain of energy.

Later, we tramp through dusty back roads and lush green fields of tobacco to reach the farm where we are educated in the art of tobacco growing, and the finer art of rolling a cigar. And of course, we must try those cigars ourselves. I am particularly proud of myself, hefting a newly rolled cigar to my lips. "It's excellent!" I exclaim, as the plume of smoke rolls out of my mouth.

Art abounds, from fantastic museums, to the back alleys and narrow neighborhood streets that only a local would know. Art spills out onto the sidewalks, and mosaics of larger-than-life fantastical figures, both human and divine, forming a community with a landscape of color that is unrivaled. From the miniature scenes, to the enormous wall size hearts made of tiny mosaics, we are dazzled by it all. I stand under the Beatles' Yellow Submarine painted on a wall that borders an ordinary neighborhood street. A friend snaps my photo in front of that painting while I'm humming, "We all live in a Yellow submarine, Yellow submarine, Yellow submarine…" I am reliving my college days, feeling the freedom, the joy of music, and being with close friends.

During this trip to Cuba, I take one afternoon to be by myself and not join the group activity. I am sitting outside reading on the patio of my casa, when suddenly I feel the powerful presence of my grandmother, Frieda, and hear her voice saying, *"Go get your journal and start writing."*

I am shocked by her voice, and quickly put down the book I am reading. I go retrieve my journal, then sit back down on the patio.

I am reminded of the first time Frieda came to me in 2005, when I began to immerse myself in spiritual studies and was doing my own healing work from my divorce. Prior to that, I had never had any experience of Frieda in my life, nor any experience of her from the spiritual plane. Her presence that first time, and now here again in Cuba, is palpable and powerful – even though it's 13 years later. I feel the depth of her words and am moved to tears. And of course, I am thrilled and not surprised that she has shown up in Cuba, the birthplace of my mother and the place where Frieda hoped to make a new start in life. My tears also flow because I feel the presence of my mother in the background.

What ensues is a whole download of messages from Frieda, as she assures me with these words: *"Yes, you are to write the book about your mother. I will be guiding you. And your mother wants you to write the book, and she will be guiding you also."* I sit, writing furiously, and crying simultaneously at the emotional impact of these messages.

I had thought of writing this book about my experience of my mother's Alzheimer's disease for years, but had not actually started working on it. I write a bit most mornings while in Cuba, and continue writing every day for several weeks after returning home to California. This experience marked the beginning of a whole new relationship with this grandmother, whom I had never met, and knew little about other than my mother's snippets of stories about her. My mother had erased Frieda from her consciousness, and I did likewise when I was growing up.

Then, in January of 2019, I return to Cuba with Barbara and Marcus, the same two friends I traveled with on my first trip to the island the year before. They are again leading the tour and the group is primarily made up of people from the East Bay of the San Francisco Bay Area.

I wanted to return to Cuba as this tour is going to the eastern end of the island, starting in the city of Holguin. Camaguey, the city where my mother was born, is not too far from Holguin – about 125 miles. Two days before the beginning of the tour, a couple of other close friends, Sherry and Lesley, join me. We fly into the city of Camaguey, in the central part of Cuba, where Javier, my tour guide from the year before, is to pick us up at the airport.

I expect a smooth arrival and check-in, but the experience is anything but easy for me. Sherry and Lesley have no problem, and sail easily through immigration and customs. I am held back, passed from one customs agent to another, questioned about why am I in Camaguey, and where am I staying. My passport is scrutinized carefully. I become increasingly anxious as I watch Sherry and Lesley move quickly to the front exit doors.

I assure the agents that our tour guide, Javier, is waiting for us out front. Because Javier had made the arrangements for our casa, I do not know where we are staying, and cannot answer that question. I am not dealing with familiar American customs agents, and don't know the unstated rules, but I am aware that I am in a Communist country, and I start to feel worried and very unsure of my safety. After much questioning, I am finally allowed to pass through.

The only thing I could think of that might have raised questions for them was, why is this American woman returning to Cuba only one year after her first visit? And why has she flown into Camaguey? Most tourists fly into Havana. What is she really up to? I will never know the reason for their concerns. The one obvious answer that might have soothed them would have been for me to tell them my mother was born in this city, thus establishing her Cuban roots. That explanation never occurred to me. I was simply too anxious to be able to think rationally.

Once I get outside and join Sherry and Lesley, I am frantically looking for Javier, but do not see him. This brings back the anxiety I thought I had just escaped. Suddenly a handsome man approaches us, and in broken English, asks if we need a ride. Thinking he is simply trying to drum up business, I say "No, gracias." We keep waiting and I continue to search the crowd looking for Javier, my shoulders and stomach tightening and becoming more tense by the minute. A few minutes later, the same man returns and manages to explain that Javier has sent him to pick us up and take us to our casa. I look at this man with the biggest relief and want to hug him. We arrive at the casa, and Javier is there to greet us. It is only then that I can finally relax.

Javier was our private tour guide for two days before we all joined up with the rest of the tour group in the nearby city of Holguin. My two friends, Sherry and Lesley, and I are all connected through having worked for several years with the same spiritual teacher, Charles McCall, now deceased. The three of us are all sensitive to subtle energetic fields and found that from the moment our journey began, we were immersed in the energies of our mothers. Lesley had lost her mother to Alzheimer's twelve years before, and though she had grieved in stages as her mother declined over ten to fifteen years, Lesley had never grieved that loss upon her death.

Interestingly – though unfortunately – when Lesley arrived at the airport in Miami to meet Sherry and me, she fell and injured her right knee and was in pain during the entire time in Cuba and limited in her walking. As it so happens, Lesley's mother had struggled from the time she was a young woman with an impaired right knee, which impacted Lesley's childhood and developmental years. Lesley brought along a cane which she thought someone on the trip might need. It turned out she was the one who needed that cane throughout our stay in Cuba. Lesley's experience was only one of many riveting connections to our mothers that we felt during our trip.

Sherry does not have children and discovered when she got to know Javier, our charismatic, handsome tour guide, that he was carrying a "son" energy for her. Her internal guides told her to *"Enjoy Javier as if he was the son you didn't have."* Sherry's mother had traveled to Cuba and had fallen in love with the vibrancy, the music and the dancing. No accident that Sherry herself, had prepared for this trip by taking salsa lessons for several months prior to our trip, and was obsessed with salsa music and dance.

What began as a journey to Camaguey for me to trace the Cuban roots of my grandmother and mother, became a powerful two and a half days for all three of us to connect to the energies of our mothers. It was as if we were in an alternate reality, one that bathed us in color, music and sensuality, as well as family and ancestral energy. When we walked into the casa Javier had arranged for us to stay in, it felt like we had come home to family, which included a middle-aged couple, and the mother of the woman in that couple. Soon after arriving there, we were seated at their outdoor patio table for dinner, where food and drink filled the table. The couple related to Javier as if he was their son, and we became extended family. The grandmother doted on Lesley with her injured knee and brought her healing remedies. I relaxed and began to feel like I had arrived at last for a most auspicious journey.

One particularly intimate and special experience took place the day after our arrival when we were out to lunch with Javier. Because he had quickly come to feel safe and loved in the presence of the three of us, he allowed himself to become very vulnerable and shared the burdens and stresses he was carrying. Those troubles included having to let go of supervising numerous workers at his house in another city who were building and transforming his home into a type of Airbnb. It meant trusting his wife to supervise those workers and to know what needed to be done, all while he was embarking on leading another tour of twenty Americans across half of Cuba. He was also stressed with needing to find ten beds as well as bathroom fixtures for the house. Procuring such items in Cuba is no small feat. There is no Home Depot or mattress store to drop into and order such things. That meant he had to do some wheeling and dealing to find what he needed, then carefully arrange for them to be delivered to his home. Rationing and wheeling and dealing for what a businessman needs is a way of life in Cuba. In many ways, our tour group was removed from the daily grittiness of Cuba, where sometimes there is not enough food, where people work hard to scrape by, and where stores often have few supplies.

Javier also shared the pain of being away from his two young daughters and his beautiful wife with whom he was obviously deeply in love. Javier allowed the three of us to provide energy healing to him, following the lessons from our teacher, Charles McCall. When it was complete, Javier's whole body and energy field radiated more vibrantly. We then talked with him to help strategize how to manifest the things he needed. That included learning to "let go" instead of trying to *make* things happen, and altering his vision from one of constant struggle to the possibility of operating with a sense of ease and peace.

While in Camaguey, I was able to locate the church where my grandparents, Frieda and George were married. A cousin in California, the daughter of my uncle Howard, my mother's brother, had sent me a copy of their marriage certificate. And with the help of Javier, we were able to locate this church, Iglesia Bautista, built in 1904. Frieda and George married there in 1909. I stood in front of the plain looking church and had chills running up my spine, knowing that my grandparents, whom I never laid eyes on, had been married in this very place.

It was a fairly ordinary church, and I suspect that perhaps the only original parts were the large arched and leaded windows as well as the exterior. The three of us and Javier entered the church. I felt the power of the generations who had gone before me. Sitting on a pew inside was a moving experience as I felt all my ancestors there with me. The place was crowded. As I sat in the pew, I felt I had almost been transported back to the moment of my grandparents' marriage vows. I felt the presence of love, the connection to the Divine, and my wonder and gratitude for my existence as a result of this union between my grandparents. Sherry and Lesley also felt the strong energies in the church and were very moved. Unfortunately, we were not able to connect with the staff to find out more about the history of the church.

Later as I relaxed and went into meditation after visiting the church, I received this message from my grandmother Frieda:

*"Thank you for bringing me to this beautiful city! This was my new beginning, what I hoped would be magical, adventurous, and would spark new sides to myself that I had never expressed before. Being in the church with you today put me in touch with those dreams and hopes. I was swept away in the moment by Cuba, by its sensuality and beauty. I well remember the winding streets, the music, the laughter, the color that was reflected in the buildings, the land, and the people. It was everything that my family was not – the freedom, the freedom to explore and express myself in all aspects of creativity, musicality and sensuality. It was all intoxicating to me, like being on another planet! My work kept me grounded though, as I was working for an important medical research lab as an interpreter. It was important work at the time, as we were focused on the eradication of tropical diseases."*

On another day in Cuba, my grandmother related these thoughts to me:

*"I wanted to escape the confines of American life that expected me to raise children, run a household, be true to a husband and lose myself to him. Though I held my father in the highest esteem and admired his tenacity, his brilliance, his ability to connect easily with people, his wide-ranging knowledge of so many subjects, I felt lost in his shadow and wanted to make my own mark. Cuba provided that exotic flair, far enough away to be removed from American strictures, yet close enough for me to escape back to the U.S. if things didn't work out in Cuba. I longed to travel the world, and Cuba seemed a good place to start. It was my father who had connected me to the work with Abbott Laboratories and I was grateful to him.*

*When I first arrived, I was giddy with the colors, the scent of tropical flowers, the freewheeling abandon with which the women expressed themselves. They were beautiful and sexy. I was caught up in the enticing scintillation of it all. And yet, my rigid Christian upbringing kept me locked into my family's strict rules that I had adopted and bought into, rules that constrained me yet somehow made me feel safe. A part of me longed to break free, but my own internal restrictions combined with the conformity of the times prevented me from breaking free. I always felt this tug and pull and never resolved it in my lifetime. I did not abandon God and my beliefs, but started questioning everything I had been taught."*

As I continued quietly meditating, Frieda gave me more insights into what led her to abandon her children:

*"Mothering became like a burden to me, adding even more rules, demands and constrictions to my tightly defined world. Yes, your mother, Ada, was a very sweet being. And on some level, I didn't feel like I deserved her, and I knew that she needed and deserved far more love and nurturing than I was capable of giving. Howard, (Frieda's third child) was a ball of masculine energy that was simply too much for me. My children demanded so much of me that I didn't have, and didn't want to learn. I felt I would be giving up part of myself. So yes, I became quite self-centered. But the act of giving up my children brought on torment in my later life that I sought to run away from in a variety of ways – through relationships with men, through immersing myself in my work. But I also attempted to fall within the guidelines of my Christian upbringing, and yet I failed in that as well, not holding to the*

*pious and Godly strictures that my parents had bestowed upon me. I always held my mother as an ideal to follow, yet could never live up to her high standards."*

For the rest of our stay in Cuba, I feel the presence of my grandmother, reveling in the energy of sensuality and color that radiates throughout the city of Camaguey – and thrilled to have her granddaughter directly experiencing this world where people move their bodies easily, their hips swaying to musical rhythms.

Our final night of the trip was the crown on two weeks of delight and adventure. Atop a tall building in Havana, a long table was laid out for all of us. The evening began with mojitos and wine flowing and salsa dancing. We let our wilder selves out to play, and it was glorious, fun and sexy! The twinkling lights of Havana cast a magical spell over us.

We then sat down to a spectacular feast that included three very large whole, baked white fish, each about two feet long, tender and flaky melt-in-the mouth. This meal had been specially prepared by our tour guide Javier's good friend and chef extraordinaire, Jorge. But the most extraordinary thing was the verbal acknowledgment and love that each participant of our tour showered upon Javier, who had been responsible for every magical step of this trip. The outpouring of genuine deep love and appreciation had many of us, including myself, in tears.

As the night wore on, I sat and listened to people in our group express their deepest gratitude and heartfelt connections to Cuba and its vibrant, resilient people. As I stood to express my own feelings about the uniqueness of this adventure, I was overcome with the depth and breadth of relationships that for me extended back two generations – back to my own newly discovered grandmother, a woman I had never known but with whom I now felt a kinship and bond. I had never realized what an important missing connection this was. And in turn, it gave me a whole new dimension to my relationship with my own mother. My mother became a whole, multi-faceted person for me, not just my mother. I was overcome with tears of joy and gratitude. My heart was experiencing a healing.

# CHAPTER 9

# Reconnecting the Hearts of My Mother and Grandmother

As soon as I was seated on the plane to return to the U.S. after my 2019 trip to Cuba, I went into meditation and internally said these words to my grandmother, Frieda: *"Thank you, thank you for guiding me here."* Instantly I felt her response pulsing through my whole body and being as she responded: *"No, thank YOU. Thank YOU for bringing me here. The love you experienced has already rippled back through the generations of our family and come back down to heal your own family of origin."*

I broke into tears, as I felt the wave of love wash over me, and felt the power of that healing love. The tears flowed, and my heart swelled with gratitude and wonder.

After being held in such a loving cocoon during my entire second trip to Cuba, returning to the U.S. was a very rough landing. Compared to the colorful, vivacious, and loving environment of Cuba, this country felt harsh and hard, particularly given the transformed political landscape of the presidential administration at that time. People here often do not connect from the heart, the pace feels unbearably pushed and stressed, and there is not enough connection between people and the natural environment of the earth. The endless pursuit of money and material things feels like the constricting wrappings of too tight pants and shoes. I missed the laughter and easy smiles, the swaying hips and infectious beat of the salsa music. For the entire first week after my return, I went into a state of depression and found it difficult to even get out of bed. I had traveled many times to many countries in the world, but this time was the hardest landing I had ever experienced upon returning to the U.S.

One thing that helped lift my spirits and the re-entry to California was a project suggested by one of the members in our group from the Cuba trip. We were each invited to contribute something creative to a collection that would be put together to remember our trip, and distributed to us at a future gathering. The writing of these poems came easily to me.

# YO SOY CUBANA! (I Am Cuban)

Oh Cuba! Your fiercely beating heart
Has wrapped me tight in your embrace.

I feel your swaying hips
Singing to my guarded hip replacement hip
      Let go! Let go!
      Claim your essence!
      Claim your God Given
      Feminine rounded body!

Let Go!
Come here with my embrace
And let me show you
The Real Cuba
The beating heart of passion
Reflected in Fuchsia Orchids
And belted out songs of 85-year-old legends
In boozy bars
Where Rum, mojitos and cigars
      Are King!

Reflected in Bright Pink, Turquoise and Green
      Cruiser cars of the 50's
Sleek lines kept sleek
Like my women!

Reflected in salsa atop roofs
And gourmet food atop
Gourmand eateries
And the mojitos flow
And the hips sway and undulate
Passion ignited

(Jealousies lurking)
Guard the door, careful
Who you let in.

But welcome All of Them
With open Arms and Hearts!

My Cuba!
Yo soy Cubana!

## THROUGH THEIR EYES

Color dances off the walls
In a spiral of life
Celebrating all that is
Joy reverberating
Between Cuban drumbeats
On a street overflowing
With dancing sensuality

Beautiful bodies
Children chasing one another
In gales of laughter
Hide and seek the world over
We walk through those streets

Stranger, obvious tourists
Yet enveloped in curious Love,

We want to know you
We want what you have.
Take all that I have
It isn't much
You in your finery.

## HAVING ALL AND NOTHING

Circle of Love
Circle of Ecstasy
Arms reaching out to embrace

The Cuban experience
Swept us up in waves of Love
Alternating with Jolting Bus rides

And Cuban pleading faces
Begging for anything we could give

No medicine
Bring it
No clothes
Bring them
No makeup or nail polish
Bring it

Colliding with hearts more full
    Of Love
Than we have probably ever felt.

We Americans, rich in materials
We seek that Heart

That we fleetingly felt Wrapped
    Around us

Showered with care, loving tears
And "We don't understand your country!"
    Neither do we.

The vibrancy, the beat
Dances off the walls
And onto our feet and hips.

We touch our sensuality
For a moment
Unlike Cubans who walk in it
Every moment and Sway
With the rhythm of Life

Made difficult by American laws
We don't understand

But we do understand
The language of the Heart,
So open and vulnerable
So ready to break
So ready to give, and give more
    We are you
    You are us
    We are One.

◆

Having received separate channeled communications from both my mother and my grandmother while in Cuba and after my return home, I had a new relationship with my grandmother that did not previously exist. I wanted to experience both women together as a unit, and to know how they might relate to each other in the spirit world. I wanted to know if a healing had occurred between them, and if they had discovered what their life lessons with each other on earth had been about.

One day I went into meditation and asked for both of them to be in communication with me. I received these insights from them:

My mother Ada: *"I never knew this woman (Frieda, my grandmother). I had no space, no place in my heart to know her. I am grateful you brought us together. I have learned so much about my family, my mother, and the forces that caused her to arrive at a very dark place of thinking she had to abandon me, Howard and Helen in order to find herself, retrieve herself, stay sane. In those days, very little was understood about child psychology, child development, and the impact of parenting. A child was seen as a commodity, a worker, a holdover from the age of child labor and the need for large armies of farmworkers. My mother had a career, and a brilliant mind, and felt the walls closing in on her as she faced the raising of three young children alone, with no husband or partner and no family. She had cut herself off from her family and felt judged and ostracized by them, even though she was the one who took herself away. She could not bear facing her father or mother, feeling that she had failed them. Her father had been responsible for procuring the job in Cuba, and now she had nothing to show for it. She and other Americans had to leave suddenly (due to unstable political conditions) which only added to the burden of marriage she was already feeling. She and my father, George, had been at each other, arguing incessantly before they ever left Cuba. The sultry, sexy climate that pervaded Cuba had spawned their hot love and passion, and fueled the dreams of an exotic life in Cuba, and perhaps elsewhere. It was the antidote to constricting rules of American life in the early 1900's. It represented escape, adventure and a life out of the ordinary.*

*"As I have learned about the complexity of my mother, and the difficulties she faced, I have more compassion for her. She was ahead of her time. She was a linguist, a learner, a historian, a teacher. No, she wasn't a pianist as she resisted taking on that mantle from her mother. But those gifts for music and piano in particular, were passed onto me, and in turn to my children."*

My grandmother Frieda: *"Yes, my heart was closed. After I was so devastated by the philandering, the cheating of my husband,*

*and the lack of having a parenting partner in him, I tried to escape back to the U.S. Philadelphia represented my cerebral pursuits and accomplishments. But my heart had closed to love. I compartmentalized that marriage as a big mistake, but drew into myself, into my mind. It so cut me off from my heart and humanity, and I didn't know how to escape. It was like falling down the rabbit hole in Alice in Wonderland. The further down I fell, the more closed my heart became.*

*This is why I came to you, Marilyn, and told you that you <u>must</u> open your heart while healing from your divorce. You were in danger of closing your heart in a similar way as me. I am glowing and grateful and proud to see that you have not done that!"*

My mother Ada: *"Whereas my mother escaped into her head, her intellect, I did that as well, but my heart was still open, to life, to love, to my children. The Alzheimer's took me into a very dark, terrifying place. However, I now see that my heart had been closed to my mother and my father. When you create that kind of closed off heart, it closes off the connection to the mind."*

And here, I see the connection to me, Marilyn, as I made this declaration to myself at age fourteen: "I do not want to lead an ordinary life. I don't want to marry, live in the suburbs, have two kids and two cars." That housewife image terrified me. I did want to eventually marry, but it was not my priority. Establishing my career was my main goal and only in my mid-30's did I become focused on marriage. My out of the ordinary life took the form of sailing the oceans for six years on a 37-foot sailboat with my husband. My life has not been ordinary, and I have had extraordinary adventures, travels and experiences.

At the same time, many aspects of my life, however, have been quite ordinary, like anyone living the ups and downs of family, work, relationships and all that life offers.

I am grateful not only for discovering the connections to my mother and grandmother, but also for the emergence of a new relationship with my father through all the years of my mother's Alzheimer's. It was extremely difficult for him in the beginning of my mother's disease as he was faced with losing his life partner, and witnessing her steady decline day by day. It is a journey of daily grieving. I think my mother had Alzheimer's for perhaps twelve to fifteen years. But she had long plateaus where she remained stabilized at each level. Even for myself, it was easy to think, well, now she won't deteriorate further, she'll remain at this level, even though I knew intellectually that that was not true.

Coming to grips with this reality brought me face to face with the stages of my own grief, losing the mother I had known, while accepting the changes I witnessed as a part of the journey into the unknown. It was that unknown that felt like a dark abyss. Yet, I was grateful for sharing this downward spiral with my father, and became comfortable with my new role as his confidante. At least we were on this journey together, though I could never know the depth of his sorrow.

How often does a window such as the one offered by my mother and grandmother open to us? I am so grateful for this window that not only connects the threads of my ancestors to my own family of origin, and to me, but one that offers healing to my heart as well. To lose my mother over so many years was to continually and gradually watch her disappear, saying goodbye over and over, and never knowing who she would be each next time I saw her. I can't imagine the depth of loss my father felt, facing this goodbye every day. What I am left with however, is admiration for the resilience of my parents as they navigated this uncharted ocean day by day, and the bond of love that carried them over these turbulent waters. And, I am also left with an appreciation of my heritage, the strength of my family, and my heart that is willing to take risks, see into the unknown, and embrace the beauty of life.

Out of these experiences, I have a new relationship with my grandmother, Frieda, one where I can internally call on her at any time, and one where she is a fully realized, multi-faceted human being, not just the self-centered narcissist that I heard about in my childhood. For this I am grateful. Though there are things about her and her actions that I will never fully understand, my heart has opened to her. I try to understand her from a much broader perspective that includes the negative forces of her time, the demons of her own mind that she must have wrestled with, as well as her being the product of a strict religious family and how that all shaped her.

I also have a new relationship with my mother, whose valiant journey with her Alzheimer's disease has spurred me to lead as healthy a life as I can, from eating a nurturing diet and exercising my body, to stimulating my mind with books and taking online courses, while continuing my private therapy practice, and maintaining supportive and loving relationships and friendships. I am so grateful for the general ease of managing my mother in her disease and sharing in much laughter, playfulness and light heartedness with her, an experience that taught me to truly be in the moment. This is not always the case, however, as many patients with Alzheimer's exhibit extremely difficult, angry and even violent behavior. My gratitude is the counterbalance to the difficulty of living through this experience of Alzheimer's with my mother and family, a sense of gratitude that teaches me to treasure each and every moment of this precious and fragile life…and to keep my heart open.

# Alzheimer's Information and Resources

**A-STAGES OF ALZHEIMER'S**

**B- B-SIGNS OF ALZHEIMER'S**

**C-CAN ALZHEIMER'S BE PREVENTED?**

**D-TIPS FOR CAREGIVERS**

**E-ON HEALING AND OPENING THE HEART**

**F-RESOURCES**

## A-STAGES OF ALZHEIMER'S

There are three main stages of Alzheimer's, mild, moderate and severe. However, some sources outline a more detailed development of seven stages, which I will not go into here. The length of each phase of the continuum is influenced by age, genetics, gender, and family history. Age is the greatest risk factor.

In the following outlined stages, I have included examples of my mother's behaviors.

**Mild**: In this stage of the disease most patients are able to function independently but likely require assistance with some activities to remain safe and fairly independent. They may be able to drive, work and participate in favorite activities. They may have difficulty remembering recent conversations, names or events. They may ask the same questions over and over, and increasingly need to rely on memory aids such as reminder notes or electronic devices, or family members for things they used to handle on their own. They may find it hard to complete daily tasks. They may have difficulty organizing a grocery list or remembering the rules of a favorite game. One of the most common signs of Alzheimer's, especially in the early stage, is forgetting recently learned information.

People in this stage of the disease may experience changes in their ability to develop and follow a plan or work with numbers. They may have trouble following a familiar recipe or keeping track of monthly bills and difficulties following or joining a conversation. It's also possible that they will withdraw from hobbies, social activities or other engagements. They may struggle with vocabulary, or have trouble naming a familiar object. Misplacing things – and being unable to retrace their steps to find them again – can also occur during this stage of the disease. They may exhibit decreased or poor judgment or decision-making, for instance, in dealing with money or self-grooming. Apathy and depression are other common early symptoms. Early symptoms can also include confusion with time or place. People with Alzheimer's can lose track of dates, seasons and the passage of time. Sometimes they may forget where they are or how they got there.

It is fairly easy in this stage for patients to "pass"– that is, to seem normal – for a long time without Alzheimer's being detected or suspected. This blind spot about mild stage Alzheimer's can also be attributed to the fact that family members are often reluctant to admit to evolving problems in their loved ones. Or, they may be unable to see these problems if family members do not interact with each other on a regular basis. Instead, memory problems or other issues experienced by a loved one might be chalked up to forgetfulness, or normal age-related behaviors.

My mother's symptoms:

*As I have referenced earlier, in this stage my mother often said, "I feel like I'm losing my mind." She was also not generating ideas of her own but would agree with something another person had said, and would also spout platitudes, for example, "You can't judge a book by its cover" or "What goes up must come down."*

*She also got lost driving back from familiar places, which my father told me about with great exasperation and concern, "She even got lost driving back from the hair salon that she's been going to for years!"*

*My mother took to ordering many magazines and things from catalogs that she previously would not have purchased.*

*My mother lost her ability to follow recipes and plan meals. My father had to take over these tasks.*

*Normally a very social and gregarious person, my mother became withdrawn and had difficulty carrying on conversations with friends.*

<u>Moderate</u>: This stage tends to be the longest. Patients have difficulties communicating and doing routine tasks, including "activities of daily living," (referred to as "ADL" in medical jargon) such as bathing and dressing, and they may be incontinent at times. They begin to exhibit impaired communication, disorientation, confusion, and poor judgment. They may become easily upset at home, with friends, or when out of their comfort zone.

Patients also develop personality and behavioral changes, including suspiciousness and agitation, or may become fearful or anxious. The spectrum of these changes can run the gamut from those exhibiting easily managed compliant behavior, to patients becoming violent and dangerous, where they can be combative and assaultive. Wandering away from home or walking around aimlessly are other symptoms of this stage, although it can also occur in the earlier stage of the disease.

My mother's symptoms:

*In this stage, my mother's behavior was generally compliant and easily managed. However, she also exhibited suspiciousness and paranoia.*

*One example of non-compliant behavior occurred when my parents made a final trip to Norway to see my brother and his family in 1993. A change of environment is difficult for Alzheimer's patients in this stage. Additionally, bathing at my brother's home takes place sitting in a bathtub. My mother could not manage this arrangement and refused to bathe, creating a new problem for my father and brother, which was not handled well.*

**Severe**: At this stage of the disease patients need help with activities of daily living and likely require round-the-clock care. They become bed bound and are then vulnerable to blood clots, skin infections and sepsis. At this advanced state patients often have difficulty with speaking, walking and swallowing.

My mother's symptoms:

*I dreaded the possibility of my mother reaching this severe stage of the disease where she would have difficulty with swallowing. She had already been unable to walk or speak for about the last two years of her life. But most Alzheimer's patients do not reach this very advanced stage, and often die prior to this stage from an infection of some sort that becomes systemic. In my mother's case, she contracted a urinary tract infection that became systemic. Her doctor offered treatment that would entail transfer to the regular hospital, drugs administered intravenously, and treatment extending about two weeks. I declined that treatment and elected for my mother to receive palliative, pain-relieving care, making her as comfortable as possible for the end of her life. This decision turned out to be a blessing, because it was made to avoid the worst-case end scenario. At this point, there was no quality of life for my mother, and two weeks of intravenous drug treatments would have only prolonged her pain.*

## B-SIGNS OF ALZHEIMER'S

The Alzheimer's Association is a very good resource for information on this disease – including the signs of Alzheimer's which are presented in this section. The organization's literature outlines common causes of dementia as well as its associated characteristics.

*Dementia* is a general term for a particular group of symptoms that include difficulties with memory, language, problem solving, and other thinking skills that affect a person's ability to perform everyday activities. Dementia is not a specific disease.

*Alzheimer's* is a degenerative brain disease and the most common cause of dementia, which accounts for 60% to 80% of cases. As this neurodegenerative disease progresses, it causes damage to the brain that results in neurological and physical disabilities, from forgetfulness, anxiety and inability to manage complex life tasks in earlier stages, to rigidity, immobility and impaired or lost speech and language as the disease progresses. Scientists now agree that the disease begins 20 to 30 years before symptoms are noticeable in the person affected. The disease is degenerative and ultimately fatal.

The Alzheimer's Association estimates that nearly seven million Americans age 65 and older are living with this disease currently and projects that figure to rise to 13.8 million people by 2050. Furthermore, the Association states that half of all primary care physicians feel that the medical community is not prepared to meet this demand.

Alzheimer's is only one of the nation's ten most common causes of death for which there has been no effective treatment or cure. Alzheimer's research has made great gains in understanding the brain and how the disease progresses, but there is no consensus among experts as to treatment or causes. The Alzheimer's Association's literature points out that much of the research to date has not included sufficient numbers of African Americans, Latinos, Asian Americans, Pacific Islanders and Native Americans to be representative of the U.S. population.

I want to note here that many of the following signs can be observed as part of the normal aging process, and do not necessarily indicate the onset of Alzheimer's.

- Memory loss that disrupts daily life

   One of the most common signs, especially in the early stage, is forgetting recently learned information. Forgetting important dates or events, asking the same questions over and over is also common.

   As we age, we all experience minor lapses of memory, such as difficulty with retrieving names or remembering recent activities. More serious disruptive memory loss that can interfere in life may show up, for instance, as forgetting the name of one's spouse or children, or forgetting how to operate appliances.

   *Notes on My Mother's Symptoms:*

   *My mother took to referring to her lifelong husband as "that man."*
   *When those with Alzheimer's forget how to operate the stove or washing machine, it can have disastrous consequences. My friend, whose father-in-law in Hawaii had Alzheimer's, had attached notes to every appliance giving very simple instructions as*

*to how to operate each one. These notes were very helpful for her father-in-law.*

*My mother burned more than one pan and left stove burners on before she gave up cooking altogether. My father then took on meal preparation. With normal aging, we may forget where we put the car/house keys. The person with Alzheimer's forgets what the key is for or how it functions*

*For years my parents had kept a small dish on the cabinet by the back kitchen door where they deposited their house and car keys at the end of each day. My father once told me that my mother asked him, "What are all these for?"*

- Challenges in planning or solving problems, in particular, trouble with numbers, difficulty following a familiar recipe or keeping track of monthly bills. They may have difficulty concentrating and take longer to do things than they did before.

*Notes on My Mother's Symptoms:*

*My father had to take over the payment of monthly bills.*

*My mother had difficulty with simple arithmetic and understanding a sequence of numbers given to her orally.*

*My parents were lifelong bridge players. Their closest friends and frequent bridge partners, our former family physician and his wife, reported that my mother began to have difficulty following and participating in the card game.*

- Difficulty completing familiar tasks

    In the early stage of Alzheimer's or other dementia conditions, people often find it hard to complete daily tasks. They may have trouble driving to a familiar location, or organizing a grocery list. People with Alzheimer's can lose track of dates, seasons and the passage of time. They may forget where they are or how they got there.

- Trouble understanding visual images and spatial relationships

    Some people with Alzheimer's may have difficulty with balance or trouble reading. They may also have difficulty judging distance and determining color or contrast, causing issues with driving.

    *Notes on My Mother's Symptoms:*

    *My mother was a voracious reader, but gave up that activity altogether.*

    *After getting lost driving, my mother gave up her driver's license. This is often not how it goes with many people with Alzheimer's, resulting in either the person's physician or family having to remove the driving privilege.*

- New problems with words in speaking or writing

People with Alzheimer's may have trouble following or joining a conversation. They may stop in the middle of a conversation and have no idea how to continue, or they may repeat themselves. They may have trouble naming a familiar object or use the wrong name for an object, such as calling a "watch" a "hand-clock".

*Notes on My Mother's Symptoms:*

*My mother was normally very articulate and well spoken. As her Alzheimer's advanced, she could not find words, or would stop mid-sentence and completely forget what she was trying to say, or end up with a word salad. Those moments were the times when I would laugh with my mother and say, "There she goes, speaking Ada-ese." This got her to laugh at her predicament as well.*

*She was a very good writer, but she stopped writing letters and communicating in written form.*

*At the time of my wedding in 1987, my husband said my mother, who was just short of her 75th birthday, was already not able to track conversations. I was not aware of this at the time, as close family members are often unaware of early symptoms.*

- Misplacing things and losing the ability to retrace one's steps.

  People living with Alzheimer's may put things in unusual places. They may lose things and be unable to retrace their steps to find them again.

  *Notes on My Mother's Symptoms:*

  > *My father told me he once found a head of lettuce on the shelf with the dishes, and found some forks and knives in the desk.*
  >
  > *My mother regularly went walking on a path not far from the house that followed the old railroad tracks, long since removed. One time she got lost and could not find her way back home.*

- Decreased or poor judgment

  Individuals may experience changes in judgment or decision-making. For example, they may use poor judgment when dealing with money or pay less attention to self-grooming and self-care.

  *Notes on My Mother's Symptoms:*

  > *My mother took to ordering almost every existing magazine subscription, unbeknownst to my father. I don't know how he accounted for the outlay of money for these publications.*

*A most poignant example of this change in making judgments, occurred when my mother ordered an expensive Lenox replica of a white horse on its hind legs, perhaps ten inches tall. Harkening back to her cowgirl days and attachment to horses, my mother would sit for hours holding this statue to her chest.*

- Withdrawal from work or social activities

  *Notes on My Mother's Symptoms:*

  *My mother was a gregarious, outgoing person. Photos of her at social functions when the Alzheimer's was taking hold portray a different woman, one who appears shrunken into herself, shy, fading into the background.*

- Changes in mood and personality.

  *Notes on My Mother's Symptoms:*

  *In the middle stage of my mother's disease, she entered a common personality change in which she became paranoid and suspicious. She was sure that my father and I were conspiring to get her out of the house. No amount of reassuring her that that was not the case seemed to quell her fears that we wanted her out. This change was especially painful for my father to witness.*

## C-CAN ALZHEIMER'S BE PREVENTED?

There are many active clinical trials underway that are designed to discover medications for treating Alzheimer's, as well as ongoing research to understand, diagnose and treat the disease. However, I am drawn to studies and publications that focus on an important and often overlooked aspect of our medical system: prevention. In July 2020 at a virtual Alzheimer's Association International Convention – an update to the 2017 Lancet Commission on dementia prevention – studies on intervention and care were presented, featuring the published work of 28 world leading dementia experts. That report outlines 12 potentially modifiable risk factors to prevent or delay up to 40% of cases of dementia. The authors found that nine potential modifiable risk factors for people in low income and middle-income countries together are associated with 35% of the population of dementia worldwide. Those factors include:

- Less education
- High blood pressure
- Obesity
- Hearing loss
- Depression
- Diabetes
- Physical inactivity

- Smoking

- Social isolation

In addition to those listed, these three new risk factors have also been identified:

- Excessive alcohol intake

- Head injury in mid-life

- Air pollution

The authors of the findings state that 40% of dementia cases could be prevented by addressing these 12 lifestyle factors.

There is new information now available that looks very promising and refutes the theory that there is no cure for Alzheimer's. In 2017, Dale E. Bredesen, MD, published his book, "The End of Alzheimer's." As an internationally recognized expert in neurodegenerative diseases such as Alzheimer's, he has held several faculty positions at the University of California, San Francisco, UCLA, and UC San Diego. He is now at the Buck Institute in Marin County, CA as its founding president and CEO. His groundbreaking work offers hope in what has been a very bleak field. His three decades of research have culminated in the first reversals of the disease with a protocol that has allowed patients to not only reverse their disease, but to sustain that improvement. Dr. Bredesen reveals that Alzheimer's is not one condition, as it is currently treated, but several. Each of these various conditions are driven by different mechanisms and manifest in different ways and at different ages. All are influenced by imbalances in 36 metabolic factors that can trigger "downsizing" in the brain. His research-based protocol addresses ways to rebalance these mechanisms by adjusting lifestyle factors, including micronutrients, hormone levels, stress, and sleep quality. He also explores the critical role of diet in cognitive decline.

Dr. Bredesen states unequivocally, "We know how to prevent and treat Alzheimer's now, today." His theories and work are very much in line with my own views of taking a holistic, non-pharmacological approach to this disease, as well as focusing on the patient's strengths and enduring abilities. This focus on treating the individual with dementia as a whole person with intact emotions, feelings and perceptions is so important and provides some hope for the future.

John Zeisel, PhD, is the author of a book, "I'm Still Here; A New Philosophy of Alzheimer's Care", first published in 2009. His work represents another revolutionary approach to Alzheimer's that provides much optimism and hope and offers an innovative and practical protocol for the care of people living with dementia. For the past 15 years, Zeisel has spearheaded a movement to treat Alzheimer's non-pharmacologically by focusing on the mind's strengths. This guidebook emphasizes connecting with an Alzheimer's patient through their abilities that don't diminish with time such as music, art, facial expressions and touch. By harnessing these capacities, it is possible to offer the person a quality life with connection to others and to the world.

In my mother's case, participating in her first day program gave her renewed hope and energy as she was able to focus on her strengths and socialize with other people who were also experiencing early stages of dementia. More memory care programs are being established in the country that emphasize these participatory socialization programs, as well as offering creative pursuits that can invigorate and energize the participants. These types of programs hold a lot of promise and deserve more attention.

## D-TIPS FOR CAREGIVERS

Being a caregiver is a demanding, difficult job that can deplete us if we do not take care of ourselves. I offer the following tips to ensure that you, as a caregiver, do not burn out and that you get the support you need.

- Keep your heart open to whatever experiences come your way with your loved one or family member who has Alzheimer's.

- You do not have to handle everything by yourself. Ask for support, reach out for support from fellow caregivers, find a therapist for yourself who is familiar with these issues, or get in touch with other family or friends who can assist. Caregivers often feel isolated and can struggle with depression and anxiety. The Family Caregivers Alliance is an excellent source for that professional support.

- Keep your boundaries clear in regard to what you can or will take on and what you will not. Get extra help when needed.

- Take care of yourself with time off and activities that are nurturing to you, such as being in nature, spending quality time with your friends/family, doing body work, getting a massage, and engaging in gardening, exercise, or hobbies, etc.

- Get adequate sleep, drink a lot of water and eat a healthy diet.

- Follow mindfulness – slow down, focus on your breath and breathe deeply, practice being in the present moment, even if it's just being quiet or having a cup of tea.

- Know that you are doing important work, you are called to it! And that you are not alone!

## E-ON HEALING AND OPENING THE HEART

The heart is the source of both our joy and our sorrows. Though painful experiences are part of being human, it is critical that we do everything we can to heal and open our hearts. The first part of this process is to accept that we deserve this healing, and to know that it is possible when we put our minds to it. We do not need to accept suffering and pain as a way of life. We are unique, beautiful beings of light with gifts to offer the world! We deserve goodness, health and happiness! The following are some of the things that I recommend building into your daily life and thoughts to help heal and open your heart:

- Practice random acts of kindness. Look for small ways to contribute to someone, even a smile or hello as you pass someone on the street.

- Monitor your thoughts throughout the day. Let go of negative, self-defeating thoughts that don't serve you or anyone. Your thoughts carry energy and communicate to the world even if you don't say a word.

- Set an intentional positive tone and thoughts at the beginning of the day, in meditation if possible. Develop the habit of checking in with your thoughts to see that you are maintaining that positive tone.

- Meditate or spend quiet self-reflective time – focus on opening the heart to receiving and giving love. There are many books, recordings and courses available to help you learn meditation and self-healing. "Insight Timer" is an excellent app that can be downloaded for free onto your phone. It contains hundreds of meditations, guided or not, with music or not, timed, short or lengthy, longer courses for a fee, etc. The possibilities are endless and can be designed to fit your needs. "Calm" is another app that can be downloaded to your phone, and contains many wonderful tools to help with sleep, meditation, and relaxation. It includes guided meditations, sleep stories, music, breathing techniques, mindfulness exercises, soundscapes, and stretching exercises. There are many books on meditation and mindfulness that are a good place to start. Participating in a live group with a meditation teacher, if it is available to you, can be particularly powerful.

- Eliminate negative thinking, including scarcity thinking, for example 'there is not enough _____ (fill in the blank), love, money friends, etc.'

- Get professional therapeutic support. Somatic based therapies such as Eye Movement Desensitization and Reprocessing, (EMDR), Neuro-Linguistic Programming (NLP), Somatic Experiencing, Hakomi, and Tapping are some powerful approaches to heal trauma and painful experiences that are recorded in the body.

- Practice total honesty in relationships without blaming or pointing fingers. Include the things you love, appreciate and admire about the other person to whom you're relating. Most importantly, LISTEN to the other person without comment or judgment.

- Open yourself to receiving positive feedback, gifts and acknowledgement.

- Practice deep breathing that is centered in the belly.

- Find and develop a spiritual practice, something that connects you to the Divine, to something larger than yourself.

## F-RESOURCES

1. *The 36-Hour Day: A Family Guide to Caring for People Who Have Alzheimer's Disease and other Dementias*

   Written by Nancy L. Mace, MA and Peter V Rabins, MD MPH, this book is a top-notch guide for people caring for someone with dementia, ranging from causes of dementia, managing the early stages of the disease, and finding appropriate living arrangements when home care is no longer viable. The *Chicago Sun-Times* newspaper calls it "The best guide of its kind." After 40 years and now in its 7th edition, this book is still considered "the definitive dementia care guide."

2. *Dementia Caregiver Guide*

   Another excellent source of support is *"Dementia Caregiver Guide",* by Teepa Snow, an Occupational Therapist with over forty years of rich and varied clinical and academic experience, as well as work experience, medical research, and first-hand caregiving experience.

3. *Alzheimer's Through the Stages: A Caregiver's Guide*

This book, written by Mary Moller, MSW, CAS, helps readers learn how to stay strong, together – through all the stages of Alzheimer's. It gives detailed descriptions of all seven stages of the disease, detailing what to expect, what to say, and what to do, described as "one of the easiest to use Alzheimer's Books for caregivers."

4. *The End of Alzheimer's: The First Program to Prevent and Reverse Cognitive Decline*

An authoritative and hopeful guide by Dale E. Bredesen, MD, neuroscientist-neurologist, this book synthesizes the latest science into a practical plan that holds promise for prevention and reversal of Alzheimer's.

5. *The Problem of Alzheimer's: How Science, Culture, and Politics Turned a Rare Disease into a Crisis and What We Can Do About It*

A compelling book by Jason Karlawish, a physician and writer who weaves together descriptions of substantial progress in understanding the disease's biology, economics and public health impacts, while telling personal stories of passionate scientists, political tacticians, determined families, and visionaries in care – all aimed at the communal dream of ending Alzheimer's.

6. *I'm Still Here; A New Philosophy of Alzheimer's Care*

   John Zeisel, PhD, first published this book in 2009. His work represents another revolutionary approach to Alzheimer's that provides much optimism and hope and offers an innovative and practical protocol for the care of people living with dementia.

7. *The Alzheimer's Association, www.alz.org*

   An excellent source for information, resources and support for those living with or caring for someone with Alzheimer's. Most cities have a local chapter of the Association.

www.ingramcontent.com/pod-product-compliance
Lightning Source LLC
Chambersburg PA
CBHW060435130626
46555CB00005B/2366